NEVER LEAVE YOUR HEAD UNCOVERED:

A CANADIAN NURSING SISTER IN WORLD WAR TWO

BY DORIS V. CARTER

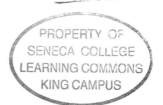
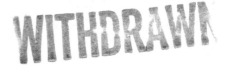

Potlatch Publications Limited
30 Berry Hill
Waterdown, Ontario
L0R 2H4

All photos printed courtesy the author.

Cover design and page layout: Thea Vandenberg

Production Advisor: Margo Nielsen

Printed in Canada by Webcom Ltd.

Cataloguing in Publication Data

Carter, Doris V. (Doris Violet), 1911-
Never leave your head uncovered: a Canadian nursing sister in World War Two
ISBN 0-919676-52-9

1. Carter, Doris V. (Doris Violet), 1911- . 2. World War, 1939-1945 – Medical care –
Canada. 3. World War, 1939-1945 – Personal narratives, Canadian. 4. Canada.
Canadian Army. Royal Canadian Army Medical Corps – Biography. 5. Nurses –
Canada – Biography. I. Title.

D807.C2C37 1999   940.54'7571'092   C99-931258-8

Preface

Amid terrible dangers, nurses and physicians play a heroic part in tending the sick and wounded, and saving lives. The Canadian medical profession has never been backwards in taking up seemingly impossible tasks in theatres of war. G.W.L. Nicholson described this well in **Canada's Nursing Sisters**, a history published for the Canadian War Museum in 1974. A first person singular account of such experiences, appearing a generation after that history, is a welcome and useful reminder that brings that danger, the excitement, and often the fun of life as a wartime nursing sister alive.

This interesting memoir is one of many that have appeared as the Second World War recedes farther into our past. Every memoir has its own merit, no matter how many are written, and the particular merit of Doris Carter's recollections is that she can tell us, perceptively and amusingly, about a world that no longer exists. The nursing profession has rigorous standards, but in the 1940s these standards were accompanied by conventions that even then, to young women of the day, were tiresome relics of a somewhat chauvinistic society.

This book will no doubt stir memories of those who were there; it certainly enlightens those of us who were not.

W.A.B. Douglas
Official Historian
Canadian Armed Forces
1973-1994

Acknowledgements

When I donated my uniforms to the Canadian War Museum in Ottawa, the staff suggested I tape my experiences for use in future Museum exhibits. I knew then that I would write about those experiences, and try to get them published as a book. For their encouragement, I thank the Museum staff.

I thank my cousin Esme Cahill of Contoocook, New Hampshire, who typed the first version of the manuscript. Without me beside her to decipher my handwriting, this must have been difficult!

Thank you to Col. R.L. and Mrs. Raymont of Ottawa, friends who have given me great encouragement — and an introduction to Dr. W.A.B. Douglas, Director General, History, National Defence, Ottawa. He wrote a letter to send with a copy of my manuscript to potential publishers. Dr. W.J. McAndrew did the same, and I thank them for their help.

Mary Raymont suggested to her daughter-in-law, Lindalee Tracey, that she use part of my war story in an article she was writing for **Chatelaine.** It appeared as "My War" in the August 1995 issue. Thank you both.

I thank Pat MacGregor, who volunteered to help me re-edit the manuscript. We spent many hours at my dining room table working on it. She then sent copies to all sorts of publishers, but they all returned them, although with very kind refusals.

I was in despair of seeing my manuscript published, when I saw an advertisement in **The Globe & Mail** for two books of war experiences — **Generals Die in Bed** by Charles Yale Harrison and **One Man's War** by Stuart Waters — published by Potlatch Publications Limited.

I thought it might be lucky to send it to them. Although unable to publish it at the time, Robert Nielsen, President, praised my book and encouraged me to keep sending it out. He kept the manuscript, hoping to find another interested publisher.

My family and friends encouraged me for the next few months to carry on, but it was all to no avail. In the meantime, a large collection of memoirs entitled **The Military Nurses of Canada: Recollections of Canadian Military Nurses** appeared, edited by Edith Landells. Finally, Mr. Nielsen phoned me again — he had decided to publish the book.

I would like to thank Robert Nielsen for taking such an interest in **Never Leave Your Head Uncovered: A Canadian Nursing Sister in World War Two.** He has spent many hours editing and revising the manuscript, and encouraging me to include additional material regarding my experience of war — even some news concerning my "love life"! (I told him initially that such information was too personal, but he would not take no for an answer!) Initially, the book consisted largely of material taken from my diaries, but in recent months additional details have been added, and other memories which are impossible to forget.

Robert did further research to provide a more comprehensive historical context for the book, including details of battles which were relevant to my experience. He also came up with the idea of dividing the book into "parts", and supplied a title for each chapter.

As a result of our joint efforts, the manuscript which I initially submitted, consisting of 93 double-spaced pages, eventually grew to 206. I sincerely hope that the reader will find it as interesting to read as it was to write!

The book as a whole is an account of my experience as a lieutenant nursing sister in the Royal Canadian Army Medical Corps during World War II.

Ottawa, Ontario   Doris V. Carter

Dedication

To my sister Eva Kingsmill, my brother Donald Carter, and to the nursing sisters who served in the Royal Canadian Army Medical Corps throughout the Mediterranean area in World War II.

Table of Contents

Part One — From Canada

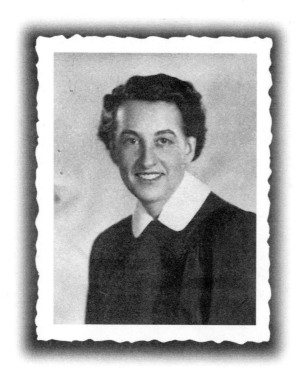

CHAPTER ONE

From Pink Hats to Navy Blue

I n July 1984 I was shocked to read in **The Globe & Mail** of the finding of the SS *Leopoldville*, a troop ship that was sunk in the English Channel on Christmas Eve 1944. She was carrying American troops to France to participate in the Battle of the Bulge, and after leaving Southampton had been torpedoed by a German U-boat, just as the lights of Cherbourg came into view. It sunk within ten minutes, with a loss of 802 U.S. soldiers, the worst U.S. sea disaster of the Second World War.

As I had served as a lieutenant nursing sister in the Royal Canadian Army Medical Corps from 1940 to 1945, reading the article brought back memories of my trip across the Atlantic on the *Leopoldville*. We sailed from Canada for England on 1 December 1940, travelling without a convoy. Because of the gourmet food we were served, we believed it was the first time the former Belgian luxury liner had been used as a troop ship. It would be a long time before I would again enjoy a dinner consisting, in part, of "Oyster on the Half Shell", "Cream of Celery", "Poached Halibut", "Roastbeef Renaissance", chocolate ice cream and coffee!

I was born in Liverpool, England, and, when six months old, came to Canada with my parents, a two-year-old sister, and an aunt. We travelled on a ship of the Cunard line, landing in Saint John, New Brunswick. My mother told us there was a terrible storm off Newfoundland, and she froze her hands in her thin kid gloves. We stayed at the Royal Hotel, and went by train to Woodstock, New Brunswick. My mother was aghast at the smallness of the town. I went to elementary and high school there, and then to the Provincial Normal School in Fredericton for one year.

I went into nursing training at the Royal Victoria Hospital in Montreal in 1932, graduating in 1935. As a private duty nurse, mostly at the RVH, I was paid five dollars for a twelve-hour duty, day or night, and often worked only six days a month. This was during the Depression, when there was not much work available. The Nurses' Registry would call if there was work; if a nurse worked three days or nights or more, when she came off duty she had to register again, and went to the bottom of a long list. If, however, she worked only one or two days or nights, she stayed on top, and got another case sometimes at once.

When Hitler invaded Poland on 1 September 1939, I went with another nurse, a friend and fellow graduate, to the Registered Nurses' Association of Quebec, located in the Medical Arts Building in Montreal. We had seen the ominous headlines in the newspapers, and decided that now was the time to volunteer for war service. We explained to the Registrar that we wanted to serve as military nurses. She was astonished at our request, and could tell us only that there was nothing organized for wartime medical services. She instructed us to leave, telephone her, and then she would take our request! Mystified, we did as she bade, not quite believing we had been registered, although she did take our names, addresses and telephone numbers.

A few weeks later I met Dr. Sandy McIntosh, one of the chief surgeons of the RVH, who told me I had been assigned to the Army unit where he was to be Head Surgeon — No. 14 Canadian General Hospital — which would be going overseas with No. 1 Canadian General Hospital and No. 1 Neurological Hospital. All three were from Montreal — No. 14 from the RVH, No. 1 from the Montreal General Hospital, and the Neurological unit from a section of the RVH under the eminent Dr. Wilder Penfield. I was originally asked to join the "Neuro", but declined as I did not like neurological work. I was still doing private duty, so was free to report at a moment's notice to the Royal Canadian Army Military Corps Headquarters in the Metropolitan Life Building.

At this time I recalled I was allergic to inoculations for typhoid fever, so I went to an allergist at the RVH and told him my problem. He advised me either to give up my idea of joining the RCAMC, or to go ahead but not have the inoculations. He said that one way to solve my problem was to take advantage of my rank; when I joined the Army I would be an officer, and when I went for my inoculations I should tell the medical orderly that I had already had them from my own doctor, sign my name, and leave — quietly and quickly! The orderly would probably be an NCO (a corporal or a sergeant) who could not argue with me, a lieutenant. When the time came, I would do as he instructed — I was an officer, a corporal was giving the inoculation, I informed him I had already had the inoculation, checked my name, and passed on in the parade. To my astonishment it worked, exactly as planned! I had "pulled rank" with success, my first experience of power. Being an officer had its advantages!

Shortly before the war I was nursing a cardiac patient who was an American. He predicted that Canada would not declare war, but would remain neutral, so the U.S. could transfer supplies through Canada without going to war itself. I was sure he was wrong, so we made a bet, the winner to receive a new hat to the value of twenty-five dollars, the price he usually paid for a hat. Next morning, 3 September 1939, Prime Minister Mackenzie King declared war. I heard the news on the radio, and hurried to work to claim my bet. Not long afterwards, the lovely pink felt hat I bought with my winnings would be given to a friend, and I would be buying a nursing sister's navy blue felt hat instead.

On 29 October 1940 I received a telephone call telling me to report at once to No. 1 Canadian General Hospital, then being mobilized at RCAMC Headquarters. I reported as ordered, where I found it was useless to try to explain to the person in charge that I was to be in No. 14 CGH, not No. 1. I learned that there were "no mistakes" as such made in the Army; I was being transferred to No. 1 CGH. I would be one of five nurses from the RVH in a group which would include five from other hospitals and a large contingent from the Montreal General Hospital.

Shortly thereafter I learned what had happened. No. 1 CGH was to go overseas before No. 14. Due to age and health limitations, No. 1 found itself suddenly short of nurses, and several were taken from No. 14. I was among that group. This was much against my expectations. For one thing, there had been a long-standing rivalry between our two hospitals. Also, if I had remained in No. 14, the staff would be people I already knew, and the management would be familiar, operating along the same lines as the RVH.

At any rate, I suspected that my new job would not be very different from the present one. I knew I would be wearing a special nursing sister's blue uniform, which had been brought up to date in appearance since the First World War. As I already wore a uniform, although of a different style and colour, this would not be a great change. And although everyone emphasized the "spit and polish" of the Army, as for shining buttons, as a nurse I was already very conscious of my appearance. I was also used to nursing patients, although I expected that the new ones would be soldiers — war casualties — and there would be no females.

It took only a few minutes for me to be inducted into the Armed Forces of Canada. I took the Oath of Allegiance to King George VI, signed my name, and I had magically changed from the role of civilian to that of Second Lieutenant Nursing Sister, RCAMC, No. 14 Canadian General Hospital. I was entitled to wear one pip on my epaulets. And just as the allergy specialist had predicted, I was able to show my name as having received all my inoculations!

All nursing sisters were assigned initially the rank of second lieutenant. Later, after successful completion of a qualifying course which had been instituted across Canada, plus six months satisfactory service, you were to be promoted to first lieutenant, at a pay of five dollars per day. However, I never took the course; later, my name would simply come up in Part One Orders with the command to put up a second pip and be a first lieutenant.

Time was short. The medical officers had already left for overseas — destination England, but not announced. I was told that I was to go with the Matron in an advance party of twenty-five nursing sisters, but no date was given. We had about ten days to buy uniforms, pack, settle our affairs, and make a quick visit to our families.

During our first ten days in the Army we wore civilian clothes, lived as we had formerly, and had no contact with the Army, except for one sergeant major. To help us carry out our new role as officers, we were trained at the YWCA every morning, where this man tried his best to teach us the fine art of military drill, but it was difficult for him to change us from sloppy civilians to Army material. I think they had plans to march us onto the troop train in Montreal, and onto the troop ship in Halifax. We had no other formal training or disciplining; we had a quick physical examination, but no indoctrination into the Army way of life or Army law.

We still had no uniforms. These could be bought only "off the rack", at Henry Morgans on St. Catherine Street — if they had your size — and the Army's advance allowance for officers' uniforms was a long way from covering the cost. We would not receive our full clothing allowance until we had been in England for a month. I had to borrow from my family to buy my uniforms, although as an officer I would eventually receive about $175 for that purpose. However, it did not cover the cost. There were three types of uniforms, each with an Alice-blue two-piece suit with two rows of small brass Medical Corps buttons down the jacket, a peplum, white stiff collar and cuffs, a leather two-inch belt with a lion's head brass buckle (that we would have to polish daily because we never had batmen), and a slim slightly-flaired skirt. One uniform was wool for winter dress affairs, one was silk for such events in summer, and one was cotton for work. Over the cotton uniform we wore a white cotton apron with a bib and straps, and the belt over the apron. My apron was made to order on Park Avenue in

Montreal by Mme. Sequin, seamstress to the RVH, who made all the nurses' uniforms. So my apron was of good quality white cotton, and fit perfectly.

A white veil was worn with all these uniforms. A navy blue suit for "walking out" was worn with a light blue shirt from Morgans' Boys' Department — really a small boy's blouse — that was difficult to wear properly with the navy blue tie, either wool or silk. We wore very smart navy blue brimmed felt hats by Stetson, with a ribbon band and the Medical Corps badge up front. Later in England we would buy CANADA brass badges to wear on our shoulders, along with our pips. We wore a Medical Corps badge on the lapels of our suits, brown leather gloves, white scarf, and brown "sensible" walking shoes. We also had black pumps for social affairs. Other apparel consisted of navy blue raincoats and greatcoats.

My greatcoat was very uncomfortable over my suit, so I approached the Major Matron to see if I had time to get one tailored to fit. I had my first experience of the reverse of power in the Army, when she informed me, "You will wear the same as everyone else, whether it fits or not!" (Traditionally there were only two sizes in the Army — too big and too small.) I realized that power and authority would come from above, and I would need to obey.

However, I had also learned that it was very easy to use a devious method to by-pass authority when you really wanted something. I decided to wait until I was in England, where I would have a great-coat and a "walking out" suit tailored, quietly and discreetly, as the Army seemed a place where things were done that way! Finally we had a large navy blue envelope purse to complement our outfit, but this would later prove cumbersome to carry with a gas mask and a haversack.

No. 1 Canadian General Hospital was not yet ready as a group; we were scattered throughout Montreal, and rarely got together except for our dates with the drill instructor. Thus we hardly knew one another, or the Matron. While the nurses of our unit were being organized,

No. 4 Casualty Clearing Station from Edmonton, No. 5 CGH from Winnipeg, No. 15 CGH from Toronto, and the Neurological unit from Montreal were already either leaving for England or had arrived. The first group of Canadian nurses had sailed for England in June 1940.

Miss Elizabeth Smellie, C.B.E., R.R.C., L.L.D., was Matron-in-Chief of all Canadian nursing sisters in Canada and overseas. There were two Matrons under her, who in 1941 would become Matrons Overseas: Col. Emma Pense, O.B.E., R.R.C., and Colonel Agnes Neill, R.R.C., L.L.D. Our unit met with Miss Smellie at a tea party before we left Canada. We were not all in uniform, as they were still not ready. Her advice to us was, "Remember you are officers in the Canadian Army, but first you are ladies. You are all gentlewomen. Your head must be covered at all times, by either your hat or a veil. Your head must never be uncovered." She granted that an exception could be made to wearing headgear "informally" in the privacy of our own mess. She also added, "You do not return salutes offered to you; you bow and smile in acknowledgement. You are 'nursing sisters', not 'nurses', and the title 'nursing sister' carries more prestige." This was a longstanding British forces rank, taken from civilian nursing. There were nurses, but the designation "nursing sister" was higher. In the forces they were all nursing sisters, with the rank of lieutenant.

We were granted a weekend leave to visit our homes. As mine was in New Brunswick, I was hardly there when I had to return! I was still in civilian clothes, and not sure whether my mother really believed I was in the Army and would be leaving Canada soon. My brother, Robert, arrived home the same evening I did, in the uniform of a private on combat action leave. He had left his second year of Forestry Engineering at the University of New Brunswick in Fredericton, and was now in the Royal Canadian Engineers. Eventually I would have two brothers in the Army overseas — Robert and Bill, who was in a Royal Artillery Regiment from New Brunswick. My brother Donald was in the RCAF, but was too young for active duty and served in Canada. One of my brothers-in-law was in the Canadian Army, stationed in Canada, and the other, Commander Walter Kingsmill, served in the

RCNVR (commonly referred to as "The Wavy Navy" because of the unusual shape of their cuff stripes). He was First Officer on *Bitter Sweet*, one of ten British "Flower Class" corvettes given to the Canadian Navy by the British at the beginning of the war, for Atlantic convoy duty. My father, Thomas W. Carter, who had been in the first contingent from Canada in the First World War, and was very loyal to England, the King, and Canada, was happy we were all serving in the Canadian Forces. His advice to me was, "Keep your buttons, shoes and belt polished, and be neat at all times. Never volunteer, or put your name to a petition!"

I returned to Montreal to tidy up my affairs, make a will, and gather the remainder of my uniforms. An odd thing happened when I went to the Bank of Montreal to draw out all my money, about $125. The teller told me he had instructions that I was to see the Manager before I did any transactions. In his office there occurred a surprising conversation. I was not in uniform, yet he knew I was in the RCAMC and about to leave Canada. He knew the departure date, but refused to reveal it. I guessed he must have been in the Militia, and learned it through his work in the evenings. He even knew my destination, and advised me to take only a small amount of cash with me. He requested permission to send the money in my account to the branch of the bank located in the capital city of the country which was my destination. This, I had deduced, would be London, and that I would be stationed in the north of England. The arrangement would be known only to the two of us, and as I had known him for years and trusted him, I agreed.

Coincidentally, several medical officers from No. 14 CGH were in the bank while I was there, and were surprised that I was still not in uniform. They took me to the Mount Royal Hotel for a drink, to celebrate my imminent departure for overseas.

Part Two — Across to England

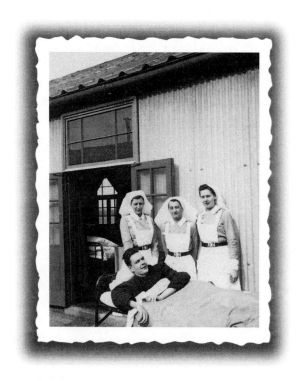

CHAPTER TWO

High Life on the High Seas

On 28 November 1940 we were given our embarkation date. Our Colonel, medical officers and other staff were already at the hospital in England, and at this time only half of the nursing staff were to go in the Advance Party, and the others would follow in a month.

Our trunks and bags were picked up, and we were left with only hand luggage. At 7 a.m. on 30 November 1940 I went to Windsor Station to board a troop train, a very long one that had started in Vancouver. Even at that early hour there was an impressive number of soldiers at the station; the train would be composed of several thousand male Army personnel of all ranks. Not until I saw that troop train did I feel I was leaving civilian life and joining the Army. I had worn the uniform for the first time that very morning! It made me feel one with the others about to board the train. A friend was with me to see me off, and gave me a bottle of liquor.

As we were officers, and officers were always expected to travel First Class, on the train we were assigned to a Pullman car, and I drew an upper berth. It was dark and cold as the CNR train pulled out for Halifax, where a convoy would be waiting for us in the Halifax Basin. I was reprimanded for having a bottle of liquor, as if I had planned to sit and drink it all myself! But I was in the Army now, and all my thinking would be done for me.

I had a steamer trunk, a small black suitcase, and a canvas hold-all, which would later serve as a mattress. (When empty and laid flat, it became three layers of canvas the length and width of a canvas cot.) I took a few civilian clothes, including a two-piece grey wool dress. Later, in Birmingham, I would buy a tweed coat, a dark red felt hat, and some clothes to golf in — before the shops were bombed.

Civilian clothes were so much more comfortable than a uniform, but we hoped the Matron would never catch us wearing them!

On the train we ate, slept, and played cards — the great army occupation. In the morning, having arrived in Moncton, New Brunswick, our car and a few others were detached from the train, and I realized we were now going to Saint John, New Brunswick, not Halifax, Nova Scotia. I recognized the area as I had often travelled through it. In Saint John we drew alongside a dock at the foot of King Street, where a small trim ship — the SS Leopoldville — was waiting for us, and in quick order we were hustled off the train and on board. It was the beginning of December 1940.

The 11,509 ton Leopoldville had been built in Belgium in 1928; her three decks were made of teak, and she had a cruiser stern. She had been operating as a luxury liner out of the Belgian Congo, and was registered with Lloyd's of London. She had also been used to carry palm oil, stored in a deep tank forward. There was a Belgian captain in charge of the ship, and an English captain in charge of the troops.

On board we went immediately to the dining room, where drapes covered the portholes, presumably to conceal us from any "spies" on the dock, and we were seated for lunch. The dining room was divided in half by folding doors, to separate officers and civilians from other ranks. Immediately we could feel the engines revving and soon the ship moved into the turgid waters of the harbour, then over the harbour bar into the Bay of Fundy. I could feel the difference, as the Bay of Fundy has the highest tides and some of the roughest water in the world.

Only one other nursing sister had ever been even near the sea. Someone said, "The tablecloths are wet!" and I answered, "It's going to be rough, and as we have no 'fiddles' (hinged rails that go around a table), the tablecloths are wet so the dishes and silverware won't slide off." The Matron then remarked that I was giving out war secrets! We were told to eat our lunch and be quiet. As the chairs were not fastened down, we held onto the table with one hand and ate with the other!

After lunch we were shown to our comfortable cabins, with two nurses in each. I shared with Jean, from Montreal. Our cabin was in the forward part of the ship and, once under way, we discovered that the heavy seas leaked continually onto our floor. Our trunks, which were supposed to be kept under the bunks, constantly slid back and forth.

We had a small Canadian Infantry force — a company of private soldiers, NCOs, and a lieutenant — on board to guard us and the other passengers. A German prisoner of war being returned to England was on board, and we often saw him walking with his guards on a closed deck. Also aboard were British officers, their wives and children, returning from the Far East. They had come across Canada by train to rejoin their regiments in England. Among the passengers were many civilians, so we were still in contact with civilian life. All these people had been on board when we arrived, waiting for us so the ship could sail at once. There was to be no army training or teaching on board ship; it would be a normal civilian-style crossing.

We never joined a convoy, as everyone had predicted, but crossed the Atlantic alone, in a gale force storm. The Navy often talked about it as being the worst storm of the war. The English captain claimed we were safer without a convoy, but afterwards we found out that the convoy we were supposed to travel with had been delayed for a week before leaving Halifax. Someone had sent a postcard to his family mentioning the name of the ship he was leaving on, thus giving the enemy news of the convoy's departure.

We sailed in a southerly direction, in a zig-zag pattern, passing close to Bermuda, where it became very warm, and the storm abated. But on returning to our northward course we ran into the storm again, now a force nine gale. The storm was so severe that the waves were like mountains, and our small ship was almost lost in them. On the positive side, a U-boat would have found it impossible to sight us.

The outside decks were roped so the crew could move around in comparative safety, although we heard a rumour that a crew member had been lost overboard one night, as well as one of the lifeboats. We were not allowed out on the open deck, and as a result never had lifeboat drill. However, there was a closed deck where we could exercise. We wore our life jackets continually, and were instructed not to undress at night. Jean and I slept in our cabin, with our trunks sloshing across the floor, but most of the other nurses and the Matron spent the nights in the small writing room, sitting up in straight chairs playing cards, probably no safer than we were.

The furniture in the main salon was roped to the pillars. We sat on the floor with our backs to the wall, or leaned against the long bar. With the exception of myself, two other nurses, and three British officers, everyone on board was seasick, but we didn't miss a meal, holding onto the table to keep from falling from our chairs! Due to the weather, there were never more than five of us at dinner — usually two nursing sisters and the three officers. These men never spoke to us, not even to introduce themselves. Dishes were smashed. Cooks and stewards were scalded and appeared, bandaged, to serve us. Our steward always advised us to skip the soup so we would not become seasick. We ate mainly solids, and drank little alcohol, again heeding the steward's advice. However, the food was truly gourmet, with formal menus showing an African scene on the cover. After dinner, the Head Steward wheeled in a trolley bearing a huge coloured cake in the form of a castle, complete with turrets. He would slice it perfectly, and the next night another perfect cake would appear. As we left the dining room our steward met us at the door with a plate of fruit for each of us to take to our cabins.

We enjoyed having laundry services, and were invoiced on a bill labelled "Compagnie Maritime Belge", and signed by the "Commissaire de Bord." On 4 December 1940 I had a blouse cleaned, which cost "N/Sister Doris Carter, Berth 62" fifteen centimes.

We listened to the BBC news broadcasts in the foyer outside the dining room. One evening before dinner we heard "Lord Ha Ha." He described our ship and passengers, and said we were doomed! The Captain then said, "No more news broadcasts!"

Finally we sighted land, and three fighter planes suddenly appeared, to escort us up the Firth of Clyde into the Clyde River. On 9 December 1940 we arrived in the Basin, and disembarked at Gourock, near Glasgow, being taken off on a small boat to the dock, and then on to the train. I was assigned with several others to an "LMS Reserved Compartment", bound from Glasgow to Birmingham. The Head Steward on the ship had offered us sandwiches to take with us, but the Matron refused. She had decided we did not need to take sandwiches, as we could have a meal on the train. So we went without food, as the train did not have a dining car. However, late in the journey we stopped at Crewe, Cheshire, and descended to the platform to get tea and buns being served by women volunteers. Middle-aged or older, they were always serving tea and buns to troops in transit throughout the war. These women were wonderful, and any time we travelled in England we could expect a smile and a cheery word with our food and drink.

But during that first train journey I vowed I would never again travel without food, whether it was against orders or not! After that, I always kept something to eat in the tin hat that was fastened to my haversack.

Part Three — Around and About England

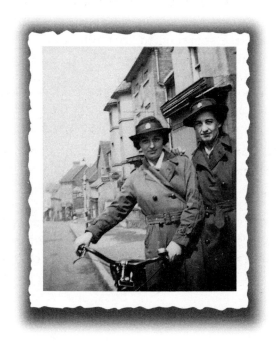

CHAPTER THREE

Bombs, Bikes, and Banana Flakes

W e arrived in Birmingham in the dark, and boarded an ambulance which whisked us to Marston Green, a small village midway between Birmingham and Coventry. While on board the *Leopoldville*, the Matron had told us that only one medical officer was unmarried, and we were warned not to be friendly with the married officers. Matters of this nature never arose when working in a civilian hospital, but she seemed to think that now we required behavioral guidelines!

No. 1 Canadian General Hospital was in the front grounds of a home for the mentally handicapped. Our large area contained a number of houses, some joined together. Three were rented by the Canadian Government for living quarters — one for medical officers, and two for nursing sisters. There were some officers and nurses who did not move in from their billets off site, as these were comfortable, within walking distance, and private. The wards consisted of a large number of long, one-storey huts, grouped in an oval and connected by roofed concrete walks. This complex, built by the Americans, was well-equipped, with an operating theatre in one hut, x-ray machine in another, quartermaster stores, dispensary, laboratory — and church. Huts containing patients had thirty beds, and were separated into medical, surgical, neurological and neurosurgical. The hospital had been opened by a group of nursing sisters I knew well, who were from the RVH Neurological Department. They had since been tranferred to Basingstoke, Hampshire, where the Neurological and Plastic Surgery Hospital was located in a beautiful high house and some temporary huts.

Two large stone pillars and a guardhouse formed the entrance to No. 1 CGH. The pillars had been erected to mark a Canadian hospital, and each bore a carving of a twig with three maple leaves. If you left through the gates and turned right, you would arrive in Birmingham; a left turn would take you through Coleshill to Coventry.

We were welcomed by the Colonel and the other officers, and taken to the Medical Officers' Mess, in a house near the hospital entrance. It contained a lounge, an anteroom, and a dining room, where we were to take our meals until a mess could be provided for the nursing sisters. Later, we would have our own, complete with mess sergeant and dining room stewards. We were given further information: as England was on double daylight saving time, this made daylight very short in the winter, which emphasized the need for blackout curtains; and, letters to Canada from a Canadian unit would go free of postage.

After dinner we were escorted to our billets, for the time being consisting of private homes. The only forms of transport, it seemed, were ambulance or truck, although a car was provided for the Colonel and Matron. Jean and I were taken in an ambulance to a house near Coventry. Our host was the owner of a candy factory in Birmingham that was being converted to manufacture munitions, mainly bullets. He and his wife were very kind, and gave us a large bedroom with a double bed. There was no heat in the house except in the kitchen, with its open grate fire and cooker. We wore plenty of warm clothes to bed in an effort to keep warm.

As British civilians, the couple who billeted us were severely rationed. Each week they were allowed one ounce of butter, two ounces of tea, and one-third pound of meat. Eggs were rare for adults, unless you had your own hens, and oranges were reserved for babies. The man and wife were allotted six gallons of petrol per month for their twelve horsepower car, and he made do with one razor blade per week.

In the morning of our first day we were picked up from our digs and taken to the hospital for breakfast — and work. It was very dark; blackout curtains were not drawn until about 11 a.m. There was snow on the ground, and it was bitterly cold. The locals told us it was one of the worst winters, with the most snow they could remember. When we arrived, all the beds were made, and everything was ready for admission of patients. All ranks were issued with gas masks and regulators, and we were ordered to carry them with us at all times, in the "slung" position. The respirator was in a haversack, with a steel helmet fastened to it, and you carried the strap of the haversack over your shoulder. We would often use our haversack — without its respirator — as a "weekend bag" when we went away for a few days.

Air-raids had been expected anytime, and they started the night I arrived. They would hardly cease for a year. I vividly remember my first raid. I had been invited by several neuro-nursing sisters to visit a pub with some of the medical officers. It was in the village of Coleshill, near Coventry. We were drinking beer in the private bar, and I was on a settee with my back against the wall. Suddenly the sirens wailed; there was a deafening roar, and crashes all around. The wall behind seemed to bend me over, and the whole building moved! Then the lights went out. I was sure we had received a direct hit. Everyone but us seemed to have left the pub, probably to go to an air-raid shelter. I would avoid these shelters, as I did not trust them — the chance of being buried alive seemed greater than just taking my chances. After what seemed an age, but was mere minutes, the lights came on and the "all clear" sounded. Some men of the Home Guard entered the pub and told us a bomb had hit close by. We had been lucky. It was the beginning of the Coventry-Birmingham raids that would destroy both cities.

After leaving the pub we went first to my billet, as it was closest. To my surprise, both front and back doors were locked. Someone suggested that we throw small stones at the bedroom window where Jean would be sleeping, but she did not appear. She was probably not in the room, but in the safest place in a house during a raid — under a staircase. One of the nurses took me to her billet, and I slept on a sofa in the lounge. We became good friends, and went to a matinee at the Prince of Wales Theatre in Birmingham every week on our half-day off.

Our patients began to arrive, victims of the raids. They were civilians, both male and female. That was why we had been rushed to England aboard the *Leopoldville* instead of waiting for the convoy — to look after the air-raid casualties. Mr. Churchill had known that the Germans were going to bomb Birmingham and Coventry by January 1941, for as long as it would take to destroy the two cities. The British had "The Enigma Machine", with which they could intercept all German communications. It was established in a country house, Churchill's home not far from London, where he could receive immediately the interpretation of the coded messages. They were decoded each night and taken to him every morning. If he had made ready for these raids, the Germans would have known he had the machine, and changed their plans to conquer England and win the war. The British knew every move the Germans were going to make, which helped the Allies win the Desert War, take Sicily and Italy, and launch the Second Front in northern Europe.

Our hospital had five hundred beds, and it was very well run, on a rigid bureaucratic system. It was also well staffed, with the Colonel as Commanding Officer, a captain as his aide-de-camp, medical officers and non-commissioned officers, and a sergeant major as head of the NCOs and privates. At the core of the unit was this sergeant major, the informal head of the hospital. Orders could go up from him to the officers and down to the staff sergeants, corporals and privates. The Sergeant Major, meticulous in his uniform, courteous, correct in all things, was consulted and respected by everyone. Each rank in the unit had his or her duties clearly defined. We were given little initiative. There was no need to think or plan. Communications came in Part One and Part Two Orders — Part One from Canadian Headquarters in London, Part Two from the Colonel of the Hospital.

The medical officers comprised a colonel, two lieutenant-colonels, eight majors, eight captains, and two lieutenants. Including the fifty nurses, amongst whom were a Major Matron, an Assistant Captain Matron, and two "home sisters", we numbered about seventy-five. We also had a dietician and a physiotherapist. The Matron was a

Montreal General graduate, as were seventy-five percent of the nurses. In addition to the five of us from the Royal Victoria, there were several French-speaking nurses from other Montreal hospitals. Several cliques formed amongst the sisters, one of which consisted of all those from the Montreal General, and another of those from the RVH plus four from other hospitals. I had quickly discovered that there were two "Sister Carters" in No. 1 CGH — myself and Grace Carter. So we became known as "Sister Grace" and "Sister Doris", and it would follow me from transfer to transfer, even though she stayed with No. 1.

Nursing sisters worked an eight-hour shift, day or night. We accepted a code, which consisted of unwritten rules:

- Allegiance to King and Country — Great Britain
  as well as Canada

- Association only with commissioned officers

- Loyalty to the C.O.

- You could sell or trade any kit or food, but unknown
  to your C.O.

- "Frank" or censor your own mail.

Our roles as nursing sisters were many: we were Army officers, nurses, friends and confidantes of our patients, and counsellors. We listened to the patients' sorrows and terrors — comforting them on one hand, and disciplining them on the other. We nursed officers, all ranks, all nationalities, all creeds and colours — even the enemy. Yet we also found time for social affairs and sight-seeing.

We were eventually given two joined houses for the Nursing Sisters' Mess and residence. The Mess Sergeant was in charge of the mess stewards and cooks, ran the bar and collected "mess fees" — a shilling a week to cover such extras as bottled sauces and extra foods, bar bills and laundry. The pound sterling was pegged at $4.44 for

Canadians, and as I was paid five dollars a day, a pound did not go far. We had a graduate dietician, with two pips, who planned meals for both patients and officers. Also in residence was a home sister, with one pip, who was the house keeper, and served us tea every afternoon. We had a complete silver tea service in the mess — every officers' mess had one. After the war I would meet a woman who worked in a building in Ottawa, who claimed that all the tea services from all the Canadian officers' messes were now stored in that building!

I was able to buy a bicycle thanks to that thoughtful Manager of the Bank of Montreal on the corner of St. Catherine Street and University Avenue! About two weeks after we arrived at Marston Green, I received my bank book and cheques directly from the head branch of the bank in London. It came to the hospital addressed to me. This was a great shock to the Matron, as all correspondence was supposed to go through the Orderly Room. Something like this needed an explanation in the Army! However, I never told the Matron the whole story, as it was my personal business. I had not been disloyal, nor done any harm. However, she was not pleased that I had contact with a bank in London before she and the other nurses received their pay through the paymaster of the unit. I was very grateful to have my own money, as the Army was slow at transferring bank books and cheques from Canada to England. One of the first things I did was buy the bicycle (and a radio), enabling me to ride back and forth from my billet in all weathers. I arranged with the orderly in my ward to keep it in working order, in exchange for allowing him to use it when I wasn't.

In the area of "spit and polish", I was immensely grateful to the Colonel's batman, who, while I was ill in hospital with pneumonia, burnt off the coating on the buttons and belt buckle of my uniform, so they could be shined and polished. I did this every night, afterwards turning the jacket inside out so the shine would not disappear!

Life was not too unpleasant, even with the air-raids, as we learned to accept them and control our fear. Our values had to change with the happenings around us. It seemed the accepted thing among Army personnel — and the English civilians — that one did not show fear, even in the face of illness and death. Here, in the midst of horrifying experiences, early learning to keep a "stiff upper lip" was reinforced. We even became accustomed to the fact that when there was an air-raid, usually at night, the Colonel would send a messenger on a bicycle to our billets, and later to our mess, ordering all staff to report for work immediately. This often meant getting out of bed and cycling to the hospital in the dark — which produced another form of fear to be disciplined. I had a light on the front of my bicycle and a red reflector on the back, but the upper half of each was covered with black paper so that only a slight shaft of light shone on the road ahead. I also had to get used to the bicycle; when I was young in Canada, my bicycle had brakes on the pedals, but my English one had brakes operated from the handles. If you went through water, you had no brakes. Very hazardous!

One night I was hurrying to the hospital during a raid when a bomb fell very close. There was a whining noise followed by a terrific THUMP. It threw me from my bicycle to the ground, spraying me with rocks and earth. How lucky I was to hear a voice asking if I was all right! It was a Home Guard, also on a bicycle going to his point of duty. He helped me up, brushed me off, found my bike and got me started on my way again, going part of the distance with me. I never told anybody at the hospital about it, as too much was happening.

The hospital had no bomb shelters, so we would put the bed patients on their mattresses under the beds, with only the bed springs for protection. I never considered this safe, and had a horror of our being hit and the patients getting tangled up with the springs! During the worst raids, we would sit under tables. One hospital hut was hit and caught fire, but fortunately it was used for storage and no one was injured.

Sometimes we stood outside and watched the dog fights, and bombs falling on Coventry and Birmingham. There were German Stuka dive bombers and Messerschmitt fighters, and we would see the British Spitfires going up to fight, planes on fire, planes plummeting to earth, and flames from the fires in the two cities. These lovely old cities were gradually becoming almost complete ruins. A German plane was shot down very near the hospital, and the pilot, captured by the Home Guard after he parachuted, was brought to us with a fractured foot. He was a guest for only a short while, after which he was taken away to be interrogated.

Later the Colonel gave up ordering us all on duty, and we would lie on our beds in the dark watching the bombing, which shook our building and our beds. Sometimes we would even lean out the windows, to see the bombing and air combats more clearly. It looked like huge fireworks displays. The Germans would let down great chandelier-like baskets of lights — called "bread-baskets" by the British civilians — so they could light up the area below them and be more accurate in their bombing.

I had an aunt and a cousin who lived in Hall Green near Birmingham. I kept in touch with them, and worried about them during the raids. After one of the worst raids on Birmingham, I tried to get them on the phone but the lines were down. So on my next weekly half-day off I went by bus to Hall Green. As I travelled, as usual I noticed the signs, such as the one often found around bombed towns and cities: "Digging for Victory." (In the stations of the Underground, I often spotted a favourite: BE LIKE DAD — KEEP MUM!)

When I got off the bus, the air was full of feathers! Blocks of houses had been destroyed, and the feathers were from mattresses and pillows, and were like snow. I had to walk several blocks to my relatives' house, and fortunately found them and their home unharmed. They always used a clothes cupboard for an air-raid shelter. I went with them to see some of their friends I had met before. They were in mourning over the death of the husband. He had retired, and become a member of the District Home Guard. He was the owner of racing pigeons, kept in a dovecote at the bottom of the garden, and often entered them in races to and from France, Belgium and Holland. Just prior to the recent big raid, he had given his best and fastest pigeons to the Government, to be used to send messages across the Channel. The night of the air-raid, he and his daughter were on fire duty on the roof of a tall commercial building. There was a terrific explosion from a bomb, and before his daughter's eyes he was swept from her side and into the air. No trace of him was ever found.

We were allowed a week's leave every three months, except during periods of fine weather when the moon was full, as this was the time the Germans did their heaviest bombing. At such time all leaves were cancelled, in case we were needed at the hospital. No matter what plans you had, Part One or Part Two Orders could cancel them. We were helped by the Red Cross, charming women who came to see the patients and help them in many ways. They wrote letters, and brought books and magazines, cigarettes and chocolate, mainly Mars Bars. One of them presented a set of placemats to our mess, enough for every medical officer and nursing sister, and we used them at every formal mess dinner. They were beautifully hand-painted with Canadian wildflowers, and I still wonder what became of them.

Some of us were invited by the Red Cross women to their homes, and we were grateful for the hospitality. One invited me for tea on several occasions, and I always bicycled because she and her husband lived not far from my billet. Their children had been evacuated to Canada before the bombings of Coventry and Birmingham. The house was a restored monastery; the floors were tiled, and in the garden on the west side there was a huge square pond, hundreds of years old, where the monks had reared fish to eat on holy days. It was now used as a swimming pool. A very comfortable house.

Another invitation resulted in a photograph in a local newspaper, under the headline "LORD MAYOR'S CANADIAN GUESTS": "The Lord Mayor and Lady Mayoress of Birmingham (Alderman and Mrs. Wilfrid

Martineau) yesterday entertained members of the medical staff from a Canadian hospital 'somewhere-in-the-Midlands' to tea in the Lord Mayor's Parlour." On a more ominous note, the same paper mentioned, "It is possible some of the barges with which Hitler hopes to invade England are being made by Frenchmen."

Our hospital was used as a clearing station for casualties from bombing raids. We sent them on later to safer civilian hospitals. In May 1941 we had two hundred and sixty-nine patients. After one of the worst raids over Coventry we received only one casualty, who was admitted to my ward — a baby diagnosed as suffering from celiac disease, because it could not digest food properly. One of the officers had been sent banana flakes in a parcel from Canada, so this is what we fed the baby during the few days it was in our care.

Later we had patients from the Army and Air Force. Many were from the Canadian First Division, who were either to be diagnosed prior to being sent back to Canada, or treated in England. They fell easily into three categories: gastric upset, low back pains, and mental disorders. Many were returned to Canada as unfit to train for battle, and often these were putting on an act so they would be returned home! A medical officer told me he had one patient who entered his office brushing himself off, and saying continually, "Darn these bugs that are crawling over me all the time. I can't get rid of them!" The M.O. replied, "Just don't brush them over on me!"

At Christmas we had trimmings to decorate the huts, and plenty of festive music, as every ward had a radio. Although officers had no social affairs with any other ranks, exceptions occurred at Christmas and New Year's. In an Army hospital at Christmas, the officers cooked and served the patients their Christmas meal, and then the NCOs and other ranks, afterwards visiting their messes for a drink in each. On New Year's Day, again the officers paid a formal visit to these messes. Officers had their Christmas dinner on Boxing Day. It was a formal mess dinner, with drinks before, wine during, and port after. Such an occasion was a social affair with its own ceremonies and rituals, and included all the officers, male and female, in the unit. Seating was by rank, and it was necessary to learn the ceremony of "passing the port"; the decanter must not touch the table once it has left the Colonel until it is returned to him. There was also a Scottish piper at these dinners — the Colonel's personal piper.

I had pneumonia that winter, and spent three periods of several days as a patient in our hospital. (I did not know I had pneumonia until I read my medical reports in 1989! I had been told I had "U.R.I." — upper respiratory infection — and intercostal neuritis.) My first bout with pneumonia lasted from the day after Christmas 1940 to 6 January 1941, after which I left the hospital as a patient and moved into the residence. With our two houses joined together, we had four bedrooms, a large lounge, a bar, a dining room, and bathrooms with baths — but not always hot water. However, I was much warmer and far more comfortable than I had been in the civilian billet. Nor did I have to bicycle the long distance to the hospital and back.

Although the winter of 1940-41 had been cold and severe, the early spring was lovely — beautiful bluebells carpeted the ground in the woods. Having a bicycle meant ready transport, and I could leave it at the little station at Marston Green and go somewhere for a few days, and have it there to ride back to the hospital — a fair distance — when I returned. Or I would buy a bicycle ticket and take it on the train in the baggage car, to go cycling in another area. I never went alone, unless I was meeting friends in London.

In our time off duty we went on picnics, and explored the ancient ruins of castles, abbeys and monasteries, of which there were many in our area of Coventry and Birmingham. We often went on bicycle trips to look at these fascinating structures. Many were religious, including buildings destroyed during the reign of Henry VIII, or during the war between Charles I and Cromwell. Kenilworth was a lovely old castle near Coventry, which had been built during the Norman Conquest. Nearby was an old abbey, a long ruin with many windows.

Several of us played golf at Meridian, a small nine-hole course kept mowed by sheep grazing everywhere, making for an exceptional hazard! A small clubhouse served teas and beer, kept cold in a stone-floored pantry. It was all very inexpensive; there were few members around, and we were given honorary memberships. It was five miles away but we cycled there and back, a pleasant time on our half-day off. A few of us were invited to go beagling with the English club nearby, a new experience. It was always raining and muddy as we followed the beagles, or sat on fences waiting for some action.

In May 1941, after coming off a 7:30 a.m. to 3:30 p.m. shift, I went to London for a weekend to meet friends, a group of Canadian and British officers and nursing sisters. We went to shows and clubs, and sometimes we were tourists, visiting Madame Tussaud's Wax Museum and the Tower of London. I loved going to Liberty's and Harrod's in Knightsbridge for a little shopping. I left London on a fast train to Birmingham, which stopped only at Coventry. In Coventry I would get another train to Marston Green, where I had left my bicycle. I should have taken the slow train, which stopped at Marston Green, but my friends mistakenly put me on the wrong one. I needed to be back at the hospital in time for duty at 11:30 p.m. The train's windows were covered with blackout curtains, and there was only one small sign at each station, difficult to read in the dark!

My plans would have gone well if it had not been for the worst air-raid ever on Coventry and Birmingham. When we arrived in Coventry, the bombing was so terrible that I could not get into the station to wait for my next train. So I went on to Birmingham. I was amazed that our train was able to start again and leave Coventry Station, because the action was so fierce.

As we arrived at New Street Station in Birmingham, it was receiving direct hits! The cavernous glass roof had collapsed on the platforms. Everyone was hurrying to get to the air-raid shelter. I ran as fast as I could to the station hotel, hoping to find help. I was in civilian clothes, and doubted I would be able to get out of the city. The hotel lobby was empty, but suddenly the doorman was there. He recognized me from previous visits as one of the Canadian nurses from Marston Green, and he could not understand how or why I was there in civilian clothes. There were, of course, no busses running. He put me for safety in a chair under the huge staircase, and in a few minutes was back with a glass of Canadian rye whisky (of which there was very little at the best of times) and water. "To give you courage to get back to Marston Green," he said. He left me again, returning to tell me he had a driver and car willing to take me! Did I have any money? Yes, I had my pound note for emergencies. It would be enough for the trip, if I could make it. We went through the kitchens to a back exit to an alley. A large black car with a young man at the wheel was waiting. I got in beside him and bid goodbye to the doorman.

The city was in flames, undergoing what turned out to be a four-hour raid; wires were down, hoses were across streets, buildings were flattened and burning. We tried one street after another, turning and going back, trying another, and finally emerged on the road to Marston Green. Not much was said, but I was back at the hospital in time to change and go on duty at 11:30 p.m. I thanked the driver. I never knew his name, nor he mine. I paid him my one pound note and was probably more grateful than at any other time in my life.

Both Birmingham and Coventry had been devastated. The centre of Birmingham was simply gone, as well as some of its suburbs. The famous Bull Ring, the marketplace at the core of the city which had been there since its beginnings, had disappeared, as had the huge building which served as the fish market. However, the lovely old church where we always caught our bus for Marston Green had not been touched.

I went back to thank the doorman as soon as I could, about a week later. He said he hoped someone would give his daughter the same help if she needed it. He was as pleased to be able to help me as I was grateful. I was never able to thank the driver again, or even find out who he was. Much later I would discover that the incredible noise of the attack on New Street Station had permanently damaged my hearing.

After that I was less eager to wear the civilian clothes I had brought from Canada despite the Matron's warning that we should not bring them. I felt that if anything happened to me in "civvies", no one would know who I was, even though I always carried identification. We were required to have the "Canadian Army (A.F.) Officer's Record of Service", which included the instruction, "It will be carried by the officer and will be produced whenever required by a superior officer." The present unit could not appear on it, but all past postings were there, each item signed by the commanding officer. So far I had only one; any superior officer could read that I had served with the "4th M.D. Canada" from 29 October to 9 December 1940, but not that I had become attached to No. 1 CGH on 10 December 1940. And he or she could also learn that I had endured 1 c.c. of tetanus vaccine on 28 October 1940, and that an M.O. had even signed his name to verify it!

Although I did not receive the tetanus vaccine, I did have an injection of typhus vaccine while in England with No. 1 CGH. The doctor who was Chief Allergist at the RVH in Montreal had told me, "It couldn't do any harm, because there is no protein in it."

CHAPTER FOUR

Under the Knife

I had become a full Lieutenant Nursing Sister, with two pips, on 28 April 1941, after six months service. This was a very easy way to get a promotion; back in Canada the nursing sisters were now having to write examinations on military matters. The promotion meant a slight raise in salary — about a dollar a day — but still did not include danger or hard living pay! We were ordered at this time to start wearing a metal CANADA badge on both shoulder epaulets.

No. 1 Canadian General Hospital was run on the British hospital plan. We had blue blankets on the beds in summer, and red blankets in winter. Extra blankets were always folded neatly at the foot of the bed. Ward rounds were made every morning by the medical officers in charge of the ward, and by the sisters. Any patient not ill in bed stood to attention near his equipment, neatly arranged, until the Sergeant Major shouted the order to stand at ease.

All staff not on duty, and all patients who could walk, were expected to attend the weekly church parades, conducted by the Roman Catholic and Protestant padres. "Up-patients" wore blue trousers and jackets with white shirts, again a British tradition. Patients were allowed to leave on a pass if they were able, but always in their blue suits.

English food was not too bad, but monotonous; if our cooks had been better the food would have improved. There was always a feeling that whenever liver was served, mail from Canada would arrive within a day or two! Could it be that the liver, which was brought from Canada in metal pails, arrived in the same convoy that brought our mail? Canned bully beef from Argentina was cooked in a dozen ways, but never very exciting; best eaten cold from the can. We had plenty of Brussels sprouts, cabbage, and beetroot. All desserts were smothered with Bird's Custard. Eggs were scarce, but scrambled powdered eggs were frequently served.

We had an attack of trench mouth in the summer of 1941, which kept our resident dentist busy checking and treating all staff and patients. As we had no automatic dishwashers, it was simple for the disease to spread, and difficult to control. I was unfortunate to have it infect my throat and tonsils, and I had to be admitted to hospital — for the fourth time. When the infection subsided, it was decided that my tonsils should be removed, and I was taken to a side room off the male officers' ward. After great discussion, I was told the operation could be done under a local anaesthetic, something I had been asking for from the time I knew I was to have the tonsillectomy. I received nembutal to relax me, and went to the operating room. I sat on a straight wooden chair, with a sister and a medical officer holding me and offering encouragement. One tonsil was frozen and removed, causing great pain, so more anaesthetic was applied to the second one, but this was not much use because the tonsil was so porous from the infection. When the job was finished, I went back to my bed in the side room. I slept until morning, and woke with no sore throat, but with a great hunger. I had been eating so little — and only liquids — for weeks. Before the operation I had spent a weekend in London, where I survived on "gin and pep" (peppermint), an English "lady's drink", which numbed my throat and kept me going. And at work, I had been drinking the juice from the canned peaches in the Red Cross cupboard that was served to the patients. To this day, I can't eat canned or cooked peaches.

A week after the tonsil surgery, after all chances of hemorrhaging were presumably over, I was sent on sick leave for two weeks to a rest home for nursing sisters. It was in a lovely house rented by the Canadian Government, set in beautiful grounds outside the town of Welwyn Garden City, Hertfordshire. The estate was called Digswell Place, and it was owned by Colonel Kenneth Maitland and supervised by Mrs. Gertrude Gilson, whom we called "Squire Gilson." She had been a nursing sister during World War One, and had married an English officer. The home was staffed by elderly women, and the Maitlands lived in an apartment over the garage. One could arrange to go there on leave, or just go down from London for the night. Bed and breakfast cost about three shillings and sixpence.

I was sent alone by train from Birmingham, and had to change trains in London by taxi, carrying my gas mask, suitcase, and purse, no easy thing when I felt hardly able to walk! While I was resting on a luggage rack waiting for my train in London, two soldiers came up and asked if I was ill, and offered to help. They put me and my goods on the train to Welwyn Garden City, with my warm thanks. Squire Gilson had sent a taxi to meet me (a very old one, always driven by the same elderly man). After my arrival I was put to bed in a small single room facing the garden, where I was very well looked after — pampered, in fact. Another sister there was from No. 5 CGH, recovering from an appendectomy.

During my second week the sisters of No. 5 Canadian Casualty Clearing Station arrived in England from Ottawa, and came to Digswell Place for a few days until going to their unit. I took them to nearby St. Albans to see the Roman Wall and the Cathedral. Squire Gilson took "the appendectomy" and myself to London for "a treat", to see **Chow Chin Chow**, a show which was running through World War Two as it had through World War One! She said she had seen it many times during the First War, so left us at the theatre and went on to Canada House to do her monthly business. She picked us up in a taxi, which took us to the train station for the return journey.

At this time the Canadian High Commissioner to England, Vincent Massey, and his wife visited Digswell Place. He would later become Canada's first native-born governor-general. The Masseys presented us with several bicycles, which was wonderful as we were able to cycle around the local countryside. On one occasion we stopped to watch Spitfires being assembled under huge green and brown camouflage netting. A pilot had told me the cannons for this famous aircraft were made in Canada, and that they were very, very effective. The field in which this was occurring was only five miles from Marston Green, and close to Solihull, a lovely town with beautiful gardens. It served as a "bedroom town" to Coventry and Birmingham, and seemed not to have been bombed at all.

After returning to duty in Marston Green, I was ordered on a couple of occasions to escort busloads of patients on outings. We went to Cadbury's chocolate factory where, following a conducted tour, we were served hot chocolate and biscuits, and given samples of chocolates, a treat for us all. Not so palatable was a visit to a factory which made bombers.

One day, high on a hill with a group from the hospital on our way to explore a monastery, I went through a puddle and began to fly down the hill — no brakes! At the bottom was a crossroads, and directly in my path was a stone wall two feet high. My bicycle ran directly into the wall and I was tossed over it. I was knocked out cold! Luckily, there were three medical officers present to tend to me. When I came to, everyone was upset and ready to return immediately to the hospital. However, I did not feel too damaged and said I could continue. My friends straightened the front wheel of my bike and we went on to the monastery. No one wanted the Matron or the Colonel to hear about the accident, in case they ordered our trips cancelled. But for several days afterwards I had extra visitors to ten o'clock tea on my ward enquiring how I felt, especially because I had been experiencing terrible headaches. However, I soon recovered, no worse for my fall.

In spring 1941 two of my brothers had arrived in England, a corporal and a sergeant. Since nursing sisters were never allowed out with other ranks, it created a stir when they turned up to see me. They had gone, correctly, to the Orderly Room to enquire after me, but I was told I could not see them in the mess. Such was the Army! But out I went with them anyway, and I also met them in London at times before I left England. Seeing them was difficult, as we were never stationed near one another, and they were always on manoeuvers. "Lord Ha Ha" once announced on German radio that General McNaughton's

"Travelling Circus" was never still, always on the move — and so it was, with troop convoys continually on the roads, and the trains crowded with soldiers.

However, we seldom saw any Canadians requiring our services in Marston Green. We were isolated from the Canadian troops; they were always in Surrey, Sussex, and Wales in the south, or in Scotland, while we were in the north of England. Although sometimes we were full, this was the reason why our average number of patients — in May 1941, for example — was only two hundred and sixty-nine, when we had five hundred beds.

My brother-in-law, Commander Kingsmill, while on Atlantic convoy duty would sometimes meet a British convoy and exchange parcels in mid-Atlantic. These would be posted on to us. Once I received a nursing sister's hat; I had only one when I went overseas, and my sister sent me a second when it was ready. That led to another questioning from Matron and the Colonel! They were leery because I had received a hatbox from a department store in Canada, but with English postage. This happened many times, always resulting in an interview with the Matron.

One of the nurses was from Newfoundland, and had a brother, who, like many Newfoundlanders, was a sailor in the British Merchant Navy. He came to the hospital several times after his freighter was torpedoed in the Atlantic. Before he was sent on another convoy, she put together a few things for him, and the other sisters contributed as best we could. He was torpedoed again, but I never found out whether or not he survived.

CHAPTER FIVE

Into the Poor House

In the spring of 1942 we moved south to Horsham, Surrey, to a hospital of huts similar to the one in Marston Green, which was now to be staffed by another group fresh from Canada. Before we left, I was sent by ambulance in a "pea-soup" fog to Birmingham Station to meet the first of the new nursing sisters as they arrived from Scotland, and take them to Marston Green.

Horsham was a delightful old town. The hospital was located on the outskirts, but we had good bus service. I worked in an old two-storey building that was said to be "The Poor House" in Dickens' novels, but was now used as a venereal disease centre for the treatment of gonorrhea and syphylis. There were a major and a captain as medical officers, a sergeant, a corporal, some privates who served as orderlies — and me. It was run on a very military basis, with formal morning rounds: patients standing at their bedsides, very neat, with all their equipment laid out tidy and clean, red blankets folded at the foots of their beds — and sharp criticism for any faults found. The Sergeant shouted "Attention!" in a very loud voice as we arrived in each large room, and continued on through to the kitchen. Treatments were ordered, and then the day's work began. Up-patients kept the rooms clean, and those who worked in the kitchen always made sure that the patients' cutlery and china were kept separate from those belonging to the staff — including our coffee cups.

Every morning one of the patients went around taking orders for sweet rolls and other snacks. The baker was not allowed in, but a large basket was lowered from a rear window with the orders inside, and then hauled up filled with bread and cakes. The medical officers — including the Major — turned a blind eye to this practice, and I had been given permission to allow it to continue. The Matron always left the Red Cross basket of cigarettes and chocolates for the patients at the foot of the stairs inside the door. She never came in, for fear of being bitten by "the love bug"!

My small office was at the top of those stairs, where I was available to all who needed advice or help. I kept records, and interviewed and counselled new patients. Canadian officers would come in as out-patients and receive their treatments and medications — and then stay for tea or coffee. They did not have to fear that either the disease or its cure would be recorded in their Officer's Record of Service. Other ranks lost pay for each day in hospital, a severe punishment, as well as having the treatments detailed in their service books.

Once after rounds the Sergeant asked me to go and see a new bed patient who wanted to talk to me. It was a sad moment — it was a young man who recognized my name and had known me and my family when I was young. He asked me not to write to my family that he was in hospital, or why. I had not recognized either him or his name on my rounds, but even if I had I would not have mentioned him to anyone. Having a venereal disease was a very sad misfortune, and not until the use of penicillin had become wide-spread was there a really authentic treatment.

No. 14 Canadian General Hospital was at Horley, No. 15 at Bramshott, and the Neurological unit at Basingstoke, all not far from us. Some nursing sisters had applied for transfers, including me, as I felt it was time for a change. Six of us who were not Montreal General graduates were sent to other medical units. Three went to the Neurological unit and two of us to No. 4 Casualty Clearing Station, housed in a lovely country residence in Dorking, near Box Hill, the home of Sir Malcolm Fraser, Lord Lieutenant of Surrey. I would remain with No. 4 CCS from 3 March 1942 to 8 June 1943.

No. 4 CCS had originated in Alberta, and the medical officers and matrons were from various places in the province. There were nine nursing sisters, five of whom, including the Captain Matron, were original staff, plus the two of us from No. 1 CGH and two others just

arrived from Canada. My new unit was much more informally managed than the first, with less formal social arrangements. There was a
constant flow of visitors from regiments nearby, and, as a result of
this closer contact, I learned more about military customs and values,
and felt more a part of the Army.

The patients were located in part of the house and in a hut on the
grounds. Nurses lived in the servants' quarters of the house, which
included a dining room with a large oval table. I had a small room to
myself, a great luxury. Other officers were in a house nearby, and the
Colonel and Matron were in small gatehouses on either side of the
driveway.

A Salvation Army hut on the road near our driveway served dough-
nuts and coffee continually to those of our unit and others just passing through. The "Sally Ann" were hospitable and generous people,
and one encountered them everywhere the Army went.

On day shift we worked from 7 a.m. to 7 p.m., with three hours off —
either 10 a.m. to 1 p.m. or 1 p.m. to 4 p.m. — and the night duty consisted of a twelve-hour shift. We were allowed a half-day off per week.
A lot of our time was spent training Canadian soldiers who wished to
become hospital orderlies. We held classes and taught them how to
make beds, change a bed-ridden patient's sheets, lift a patient, bathe
him, apply bandages — almost everything but give medications.

We ran an out-patient department in the mornings, and the sick and
injured reported in, mostly privates and NCOs from Canadian Army
units stationed nearby. We treated sprained ankles by spraying them
with a local anaesthetic, allowing their owners to walk with hardly any
pain, and they would return for several treatments. I was often alone
on night duty, and many of the emergencies arriving were dispatch
riders who had suffered motorcyle accidents. When necessary, we had
to contact the medical officer who was on call and additional nursing
sisters, if there was surgery to be done.

On one occasion, on a cold and windy day, we hurried to the grounds of the house next door to see King George VI review General Bernard Montgomery and his troops. Someone had brought news that the King was arriving and we went to the back gardens to witness the event. Also in attendance was General Harold Alexander, who would later become Lord Alexander, Governor-General of Canada. It was a very impressive sight as the rows of soldiers in battle dress were inspected by the King. He and General Montgomery walked up and down the long lines of the 51st Highland Division. The troops wore the insignia "G.O." on their shoulders, and were dubbed the "Go Boys." They had completed commando training in Scotland, and had the honour of guarding Buckingham Palace — and of being under General Montgomery, whom they all admired. The review occurred immediately before the division left England for the North African desert, where Montgomery would become head of the British African forces. Although the "Go Boys" had been stationed nearby, I never met any of their officers until we were all in Sicily, when again they would be neighbours.

At this time Mr. Garfield Weston of the Weston Biscuit Company gave the Canadian nursing sisters a club in London, a three-storey house on Cromwell Road in Knightsbridge. It had a fine terrace in back, complete with tables and chairs. We could stay overnight for three shillings and sixpence, with breakfast served in our rooms. Lunch and dinner were also available, and Mr. Weston had provided a cellar of very fine wines and liquors. It was a great pleasure for me to stay there during the first year it was open.

Some weekends I would cycle from Dorking to visit friends a few miles away, who had some hens, a beehive, and a small garden. I would take one fresh egg back with me as a treat. They were allowed to keep only part of the honey for themselves, as the bulk went to mothers and babies. An official beekeeper, who helped people with their hives, would arrive periodically on his bicycle — in a rush — whenever the bees swarmed.

I received a parcel from my sister, who was staying in Charleston, Maryland, while her husband's corvette was being refitted. The parcel contained a battered box of almonds, some pralines, and six pairs of nylon stockings, the first I had seen. Unfortunately, the oil from the chocolates had melted into the nylons, and I had a very difficult time washing it out. But how wonderful to have stockings like silk!

As I had promised myself before leaving Canada, using my newly-acquired clothing coupons I had a navy blue greatcoat and suit tailored, as well as a blazer with the medical crest on the pocket. They were made at "Moss Brothers", who had a large works in Dorking, where clients were nearly all officers in the three services. My new clothes were made from the same cloth used for naval officers' uniforms — beautiful, darker than the material I had bought in Canada — and they fitted me very well. The blazer was for informal wear, with a silk tie with the Medical Corps colours in stripes. It was wonderful to be able to wear a suit under my greatcoat, and to be comfortable and warm in winter. I also had pale blue shirts made in London, to replace the little-boy-style blouses I had bought in Canada. The Matron was becoming more and more flexible about my uniforms being somewhat different from those of the others!

The house in Dorking had a glorious garden, filled with many-coloured rhododendrons as well as black and white, where, one sunny day, the officers and nursing sisters had a garden party. It was a very large affair, held on the lawns, and was intended to return the hospitality we had received from other regiments. Long tables with white sheets for tablecloths, complete with a silver tea service, shone in the sun. We invited friends from nearby, mostly Canadian officers, and our Matron-in-Chief, Agnes Neill, from London. There were several medical officers from No. 1 CGH at Horsham; they gave me all the news, chortling over one piece: "The Matron is going back to Canada." Everyone appeared very smart in their dress uniforms, with the sisters in their two-piece blue silks and veils, "always something on your head"!

In August 1942 I had a leave due, and my friend Marg, a nursing sister with the Canadian Neurological Hospital, phoned me with an idea. We had been planning to take our leave together, and there was a letter on their bulletin board from two civilian sisters in Aberdeen, Scotland, inviting Canadian officers, male or female, to spend their leave with them at any time in their home. They sounded so hospitable that Marg wrote to ask if we could visit, beginning 10 August. They replied that they would be delighted to have us. As I was in Dorking and Marg was in Basingstoke, we decided to make a reservation for one night at a hotel in Glasgow. We would meet there, and go to Aberdeen together the next morning. Marg had her First Class Travel Warrant, but I had used mine on my last leave, so I had to pay for my railway fare and go Third Class, which was all I could afford. It was against Army rules for an officer to travel Third Class, but at times many of us did. (In addition, an officer in uniform was forbidden to carry an umbrella, no matter how inclement the weather, or to carry a parcel — although we got around that by putting parcels in our gas mask haversack.) As I was wearing civilian clothes I was allowed to purchase a Third Class ticket.

I hated the thought of changing trains at Crewe. I would have to leave the arrival platform by going up a long set of metal stairs, across a high bridge, and then down another set of stairs to the platform for my train to Glasgow. Crewe was always a very crowded junction, with many troops moving, sometimes in large groups. I would just be a civilian, travelling alone, looking for my platform, then my train, and then a Third Class carriage.

All went well and I arrived at the hotel in Glasgow after luckily finding a cab. I waited for Marg for ages; finally she arrived, but in a navy blue uniform. I was too surprised to ask her, "Why?" We ordered sandwiches in our room, and she told me her story. She was still upset. She roomed at the "Neuro" with three other nurses in a large room. One of them had a cat, which the others tolerated, and it was "expecting." They always kept the clothes closet door closed, but one night the cat got in, pulled down Marg's new Jaeger green coat, made a nest in it

— and had her kittens. The coat was dry-cleaned twice but the odour and stains did not disappear, and it had to be disposed of. Poor Marg, still so upset, because she had to wear her uniform. A sad way to start our leave, but eventually she cheered up.

I liked Aberdeen, with all its granite buildings. When we arrived at their address, we found our hostesses most welcoming. They were delighted to see us. They lived in the centre of the city, in a tall three-storied house on a street on a hill, where the houses were all joined together and were the same design. The ladies had plans to fill our days and evenings with most interesting activities. The next morning we were up early to go down to see the fishing fleet leave, a great sight. We wandered through the fish market, and went home for lunch. Later we returned to watch the fleet returning to the harbour. Aberdeen was then famous for its fishing fleet and market.

Our hostesses took us up the River Dee to meet a friend, a charming person who was also a well-known painter. Her home and garden were lovely, and situated right on the river. We met many of their other friends as well, and were sorry to leave as they had been so good to us.

On 14 August 1942 we prepared for casualties from the disastrous raid on Dieppe. We made everything available, with all beds set up and ready — but we received no patients, because so many soldiers had been either killed or taken prisoner. The raid had been staged on the 19th with 5,000 troops, mainly Canadian, resulting in the deaths of nine hundred men, and the capture of two thousand more, many of whom were wounded. A horrible tragedy.

Shortly after this, orders came from Headquarters in Leatherhead that No. 4 Casualty Clearing Station was to move to Newdigate, Surrey, between Dorking and Guildford. We were evacuating our premises to make room for No. 5 CCS. I had met some of their nursing sisters at Digswell Place, but as I was leaving the house I came upon one of their medical officers, who had been a noted pediatrician at the RVH. He was famous for his habit of never calling a female parent or her child by name; he addressed them as "Mother" and "Baby." I had not known he was overseas, and we stopped to talk. It was good to see someone from Montreal, my present unit being all "westerners." Much later, on my return sea voyage to Canada, I would encounter him again.

CHAPTER SIX

The Fate Worse Than Death

W̶e were in Newdigate for a training course, and did not set up the hospital, although we had an orderly room for the business part of running the unit. Our new home was used specifically for training Army units, and consisted of an aged manor and several large farms. The Orderly Room and Officers' Mess were located in the manor, as were the medical officers' quarters. Nursing sisters, NCOs and privates were housed on the farms, a fair walking distance away.

We had to scrub our whole house before we could move in. However, it was comfortable — except for the beds, which were solid wood, and scooped out to hold one's body. We had no mattresses, but we had our own sleeping bags; I had bought mine from a nursing sister returning to Canada. We were told that the beds were originally from the "Duke of Wellington's Barracks" in Aldershot. I believed that they had been used by the Iron Duke's force, because sleeping on the ground would have been softer and more comfortable! But we were now in serious training.

We remained at Newdigate for two months, and were introduced to the art of self-defence, learning to kill if attacked, to save ourselves from "the fate worse than death"! Our instructors were several sergeants who had been in the Dieppe raid and had made it safely back to England. We marched very strenuously every day, and crawled on the ground along a rugged course through open country, always wearing gas masks. Although I didn't wear my glasses much on a daily basis, I had to wear them for training, and one day I broke them. When I got the opportunity, I took them to a place in Threadneedle Street in London to get a pair that the Army would pay for. After that

I rarely wore my glasses in case I broke them again, although I was shortsighted and seldom recognized anyone until they were up close!

Newdigate was a lovely spot, and we enjoyed living there in spite of the commando-style training. The blackberries were ripe and we picked them and gave them to the cook, who made pies for us. We gathered rose hips in the hedges and gave them to the local people to boil down to make a syrup for their babies. Rose hips are very high in Vitamin C, and they were used to supplement oranges, which were very scarce and only mothers with babies could buy them.

There was a beautiful old building in Newdigate, the Church of St. Peter, with a chancel built in the twelfth century and a nave one hundred years later. The five-hundred-year-old sixty-foot tower was made of oak, and was very rare. There was also a striking lych gate, a roofed arch at the entrance to the churchyard where the coffin was left to await the arrival of the clergyman.

The local citizens often entertained us with card parties and teas. One of them gave me a jade brooch, and told me it would save me from drowning. I still have it.

We moved on again, to Ford Manor in Lingfield, Surrey, near East Grinstead. There we set up a small hospital, and had plenty of patients. There were many upper respiratory infections, and injuries resulting from manoeuvers. Surgeries included hernias and hemorrhoidectomies, and there were fractures and head injuries as a result of motorcycle accidents. We even had psychiatric patients, as there was a psychiatrist on staff who ran a day clinic.

The house was huge, with a long winding driveway leading up from the main road. The officers lived in one of the two gate houses. The other was owned and inhabited by an English couple; it was circular, and originally had been a toll house. The nursing sisters lived in the nursery area of the manor and slept in the guest rooms nearby, and there were larger rooms for the patients. One big room to the right of the front entrance was kept locked and sealed so no one could enter.

There the owner, an elderly woman, kept a great deal of furniture, and she came at times to inspect it, flying along on her bicycle. She was concerned, because when the Army moved from place to place we were never charged for any damage, as the owners leased their buildings to our government.

The winter of 1942-43 was very cold, and we had almost no heat, except when we were occasionally given a scuttle of coal for the fireplaces in our rooms. We had no wood to start a fire, so poured old oil from military vehicles over the coals. We threw in a match, and quickly put a metal screen across before the blaze went up with a roar. It was a wonder we never blew ourselves up, complete with house!

One morning I was on duty on the second floor, in a large room with windows all across one side, passing out basins of water to the bed patients. Suddenly there was a shout — "Sister, get down, get down!" I was pushed to the floor and the patients went down as well, as a German plane flew by very low, strafing the house. Bullets sprayed the room, shattering the windows. We were lucky that one of the patients saw or heard the plane in time for us to duck. Although no one was hit, we learned later that children had been killed while playing in their schoolyard southeast of us by the same plane, on its return trip to Germany. To ensure his safe landing, the pilot had dropped his bombs, and used his guns on anything he desired.

Before Christmas the Matron, our third since I had been with No. 4 CCS, criticized me for having a hole in the crown of my hat. It had been caused by a pin I aways used to hold the hat in place. I was told to find a new one, even though our hats were not sold in England, and there was little chance of getting one from Canada. Our matron was really not a pleasant person! Someone told me there was a RCAMC nursing sister's hat in a men's hat shop on Bond Street, so I went to London. I found the shop, and climbed a wide staircase to the second floor. Yes, they had a navy felt hat that had been ordered by a Canadian nursing sister, but it had never been picked up or paid for. I tried it on and it fit.

To get to London, we would bicycle to Lingfield Station to catch the train. Upon returning in the dark, we disliked cycling past the famous racecourse, where hundreds of German prisoners were now housed, even though the place was well guarded and surrounded by a high wall topped with barbed wire. We then had to negotiate the long sunken driveway from the main road to the manor house — a very eerie ride, especially at night. However, we never did it alone, concerned that the cows wandering on top might be more human than bovine!

My mother wrote to ask me to visit the son of a friend in the RCAF who had been shot down, and was being treated at the Queen Victoria Hospital. East Grinstead was the location of the hospital, a plastic surgery facility for burn patients, staffed by the famous surgeon Dr. Archibald McIndoe and his Canadian assistant, Squadron Leader Dr. Ross Tilley. The patient I visited was under Dr. McIndoe's care, and afterwards I was often invited back for tea. Dr. McIndoe was very successful performing surgery on the ears, faces and hands of burn victims, and was continually trying to improve his methods of replacing eyelids. He operated in a tiny room, and when it rained and the roof leaked while he was working, someone would hold an umbrella over him!

Many RCAF and RAF men were patients at the Queen Victoria for long stretches of time — a total of six hundred and thirty by war's end, one hundred and seventy of them Canadian. Patients were encouraged to go into town and to parties, even before their treatments had been finalized. In 1942, the Canadian Government gave a grant of twenty thousand pounds for the building of a plastic surgery and jaw injuries wing at the hospital, for the treatment of RCAF casualties. Although I was there too early to see it, the building was completed in 1943, with one hundred and forty-six beds, and was dedicated to the memory of all RCAF servicemen — past, present, and future — lost in the war.

The delightful people who lived in the "Round Toll House" invited the nursing sisters and medical officers for card games, and we took turns going. The Matron or the Colonel played bridge with our hosts, while the rest of us, a dozen or so, sat around a large oval table, each with a pack of cards, and played double solitaire, placing our cards altogether in the centre of the table. What an uproar! Often there were other guests: the two padres, patients from the Queen Victoria Hospital, and men from a nearby Irish regiment.

I lost my watch in East Grinstead. I had left it at a jeweller's to be repaired, but the shop was bombed during a raid, and with it my watch. Somehow I managed to get a Big Ben pocket watch very cheaply, and it lasted the rest of the war, always in my jacket or apron pocket.

On 5 May 1943 I was told I was going on an operating room course, to No. 8 CGH in the Aldershot area. I had to pack at once, pay up my mess fees, retrieve my laundry, and leave in the transport provided. I loaned my golf clubs to a friend, who was to send them to the luggage holding unit if he moved anywhere. I never saw them again.

Part Four — Down to Algeria

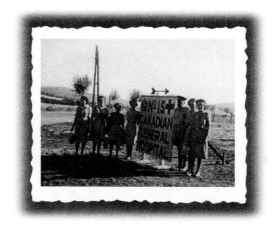

CHAPTER SEVEN

A Patch of Red

No. 8 Canadian General Hospital was located in a large building previously used as an English civilian hospital; I never did learn where their patients went. The sisters stayed in small houses at the back of the building, where the civilian staff had lived. I had a tiny room downstairs in the front of a house I shared with a dietician and a psychotherapist. Each wore one pip on her uniform.

The nursing sister in charge of the operating room had her arm in a cast, the result of a recent fracture. I did general work in the operating room, and whenever there was a wedding or other special event in the unit, I kept it going while the others attended. The surgeons did a large number of herniotomies and hemorrhoidectomies. One Canadian officer, who had lost both hands in a hand-grenade training accident, came daily for new dressings, and insisted on opening the doors himself. A very brave man.

I was also assigned to a Canadian obstetrical medical officer from Montreal — we were the only two from that city. The hospital had an obstetrical department for Canadian Force's wives and Canadian women in the military. The medical officer used caudal anaesthetic, a new spinal variety, for deliveries. I enjoyed obstetrical work, including helping with the deliveries. Once I had to deliver a baby alone in an emergency, as the M.O. was not available — fortunately, I remembered my training from the Royal Victoria!

In the spring of 1943 an order was received stating, "All Nursing Sisters will salute Senior Officers and accept salutes." This was an action bringing us closer to our desired status in the Army. Without warning I was summoned to the Matron's office. The Chief Matron of Nursing Sisters Overseas, Colonel Agnes Neill, was there, and she asked if I would join another small unit, possibly a casualty clearing station, which was on orders to leave England for action. She said she would accept the offer herself if she was in my shoes. It called for a quick impulsive decision to be made on the spot, so I decided to accept. I didn't need to be urged! And I never regretted having made the decision.

The very next day I left No. 8 CGH, and went by ambulance to No. 15 CGH at Bramshott, Hampshire, in company with a padre who was going to the same place to be re-posted. There I found the other five nurses for the new unit. They had been told as I had; we would be in a casualty clearing station, but under the Matron of No. 15 CGH. I was late being recruited because I had been on a course, so I was a week behind the others in documentation, training, and packing.

The next day the officer responsible for luggage went through all my belongings with me, sorting out the things to be sent to the baggage holding unit in England, and those I would take with me. He was sure we were going to a country with a hot climate, so my warm clothes — woolen vests, sweaters, etc. — went into storage. I would regret this later in the cold winters. I was issued with men's small size khaki wool pullover sweaters, and wool shirts, as well as a new respirator, ground sheet, webbing, and a grey woolen blanket. I was told the blanket was to wrap me in if I died! It was to be carried rolled on top of my back-pack. The second day I was given my backpack — a tin hat and haver-sack. I was fully equipped.

From this time on, in addition to the flashes of the British Eighth Army, I would wear the "Old Red Patch", the red triangle insignia of Canada's First Division, on the left arm above the elbow of my uni-forms. Up to this point my uniforms had been blue, as was the case with the others in the unit. But later I would be in khaki, and this, along with wearing the flashes of the First Division, would make me feel much more a part of the Canadian Army. And once I left England, I would have no civilian friends; they would all be from the fighting forces of various countries. It would take me three years to become socialized into my new way of life. And it would not be until I was on a troop ship leaving England for Canada in 1945 that I would realize how much I had changed during the preceding five years.

There were seventy-five of us, including the nurses from No. 15 CGH and we six. From 10 to 28 June we were drilled every day and marched long distances four abreast — about a mile the first day, which was gradually increased to several miles as we became more able. Then we had a fall-out, before returning on the march to the unit for lunch. With all our gear, our endurance exercises were exhausting, as we were carrying the equivalent of our body weight on our backs! However, we slowly became well-conditioned, and after a while found the marches more comfortable. Meanwhile, we had two false starts to the station, as if we were going to board a train — just to keep us on our toes.

I had to make one trip back to each of No. 4 CCS and No. 8 CGH to pay outstanding mess and laundry bills, as I would be leaving soon. I also went to see both my brothers, who were with units on the south coast. Before I left to visit them I had to get permission, and leave my name and destination. The train trip took all one Sunday, and I travelled on my own, an unusual experience. I went first to Petworth to see Bill, who was a sergeant with an artillery unit. They had been stationed at Woodstock, Oxfordshire, the estate of the Duke of Gloucester, but were now in Sussex. Then I went to find my twenty-two-year-old brother Bob, in the same county. I had to change trains, and get a bus, and finally tracked him down. It was difficult, but being a lieutenant nursing sister helped, as everyone guided me from one place to another. I found Bob in a Field First Aid Hut. He had been on manoeuvers, and a gun carrier had run over his foot, fracturing several bones. He was in bed, with a pair of crutches nearby, and was to be sent back to Canada! He would arrive before Christmas, and return to university, after serving two years in England.

At this time my father became very ill, and was in my old hospital in Montreal. He had been referred to the RVH from our hospital at home by our family doctor because it — along with the Montreal General —

was the best hospital in eastern Canada to help him. He had contracted spinal meningitis during the First World War, to which his present illness was attributed. I received a comforting letter from my mother, who had left New Brunswick to be with him, telling me he was improving.

One day I was ordered to the O.C.'s office. A private announced me, I entered, saluted, and said, "Sister Carter, Sir." His reply was, "You are struck off strength as of now." I saluted and left. Later in the day I was ordered back to the O.C.'s office. He said, "You are back on strength." I asked why, but he had no reply except, "Dismissed!"

It was a great puzzle! No one knew anything to tell me. But on returning to Canada after the war, a friend of my father would tell me he had been trying to locate my brothers and me to bring us home before my father died. He wanted very much to see us. The friend was a top executive at Seagram's in England, and had used their phones and wires. He located me and then was told they had lost me as well as my brothers. So that explained my being struck off strength and put back on. I think the O.C. had thought it was a useless thing to do in a war. My father would have been dead before I arrived.

Over the next two weeks we breakfasted every morning at 7 a.m., and began drill at 7:30, but we now had some free time after lunch. On 27 June we handed in our clothing coupons. These were a life saver — without them I could not have purchased a new suit, greatcoat, blazer, hat and shoes. I bought flat-heeled brown shoes in a shop in Guildford, and they sent me another pair later that would reach me in North Africa. That same day we received luggage tags, and Red Cross cards to send to relatives and friends. It was really not worth sending them, as there was little one could write without the Army blacking it out, and it took ages before they arrived in Canada. I received my new pale blue shirts from London, and decided to take them with me. They fitted perfectly, and looked very sharp with my dark blue suit and coat! I wondered why I had bothered to buy them, but we would be in blue uniforms as much as khaki later on.

We had no drill on the 28th. That day khaki berets were given out to the other nursing sisters, but there were none for our small unit as not enough had been ordered. I guess we really had not been expected! Not having a khaki beret would prove a problem for us, because, of course, we had to have our heads covered! Later in Algeria I would find myself walking up the line of nurses' tents to find someone on night duty, or not planning to go out, to lend me her beret. Finally, I would be able to buy my own in an officers' shop in Catania, Sicily, although even then it would be the black beret of the tank corps. The Matron would object, as usual, but finally give up and just not see it!

All through the war you had to be careful of the weight of your steamer trunk. We were now told that it could not weigh more than a hundred and twenty pounds, but we could carry as much as we were able. I weighed myself fully equipped, and my weight was doubled.

That same day we had lunch at 11 a.m., high tea at 4 p.m., and at 6 were paraded, loaded into lorries, and taken to Haslemere Station at 8. As we were in day coaches with no sleeping cars, we assumed we would not be going far that night. But as we continued to move, we realized we would have to try to sleep in the compartment. With four of us to a compartment, we finally decided that two could sleep in the seats and two in the luggage racks, and as I was one of the smaller ones I was hoisted into a rack and slept on my grey blanket. We passed through Guildford and Reading on our way north, then Crewe Junction, Worcester and Birmingham, before stopping at Carlisle. Here we were given mugs of hot sweet tea before moving on to Gourock, Scotland, arriving early in the morning. We de-trained and marched in full gear into a large passenger "shed" on the harbour. We had to stand until noon, not being allowed even to slip off our backpacks for comfort.

When we at last went up the gangplank of the Greek liner SS *Nea Hellas*, I was almost unable to make it, my gear being so heavy; in addition to full equipment, I was carrying a small suitcase and a large purse. I finally reached the top, and two soldiers, standing one either side of the gangplank, lifted me down onto the deck; I was so pleased to have their assistance, as I couldn't have stepped off the gangplank myself. I would have fallen flat on my face! Publicity photographs were taken, and newsreels for the theatres in Canada.

We were assigned at once to cabins; I received a "Berthing Card" indicating I had a "Mattress Hammock" in "Cabin 22" on "Deck A." The small cabin had two lower and two upper bunks, and I shared with three other nursing sisters. We were at very close quarters, with one wash basin, but we counted ourselves lucky to have a cabin. We went to get our meal cards, and were assigned to the "Forward Dining Saloon", and would attend "Second Sitting" as we were junior officers. Everything was organized as if we were taking a private trip First Class, although the portholes in the cabins were closed and blacked out.

The nursing sisters shared A Deck with other officers and war correspondents, the remainder of the ship being filled with troops. The decks were clear except for piles of life rafts, because there weren't enough lifeboats if we had to abandon ship.

In the dining saloon we had fresh white bread and rolls — with butter — fresh eggs and fresh meat. In England we had been eating a specially fortified bread with dark streaks in it. It was rather good, but seeing white bread again was a nice surprise. Great food before the battle! We were also served, before lunch and dinner, tall glasses of coloured drinks made from powder, on silver trays borne by stewards in white jackets. Some of the officers had brought liquor on board in their suitcases, and they would fortify these drinks — both theirs and ours.

The Matron read the ship's orders to us at 2100 hours; we could wear skirts without jackets, "No hats or berets" (Surprise!), and we were to sleep in most of our clothes to be ready for any emergency.

The Basin at Gourock was filled with ships containing Canadian troops. On 30 June we were still in dock, and had our first lifeboat drill, in our shirts with the sleeves rolled up. Our ship pulled into the mouth of the river, and anchored. We sat on the deck in the sun, and talked to the other officers.

Still at anchor, on 1 July we received a welcome ration of cider, and were also issued with anti-mosquito ointment and iron rations. The rations consisted of a shallow tin containing a fortified chocolate mixture, and were to be carried at all times in our raincoat pockets, but never touched unless food was needed in an emergency. We listened to Orders, which were read to us in the morning, and then spent our time sitting on top of the rafts, watching ships manoeuvering. We were assigned to specific lifeboats, and had another lifeboat drill.

We sailed at 2200 hours on 1 July. We went through the boom and out to sea, with several cruisers and aircraft carriers accompanying our convoy. We were in a long column of passenger vessels and freighters, and we were the last in line. We went down the west coast of England, and then out into the Atlantic. There were two small destroyers in our section, dashing around and about the ships, guarding us. The corvettes and destroyers were always going back to collect freighters, and bringing them into line in the convoy.

It was hard to believe we were on our way to fight a war, and we spoke often of the troops in the forward group of ships, who would land first. On 2 July Orders were read for the last time. We lay in the sun, feeling the ship rolling and changing course. We enjoyed tea on deck, and watched a school of porpoises. There was no cider this time, but iced lime — officially, no liquor was allowed on board. We were told we would have lectures the next day. We went to bed early, and turned our clocks back one hour at midnight. The sea was rough.

The next day was a Saturday and we sat on rafts until the brief boat drill. There were about a dozen rafts on deck, and they were very comfortable to sit on — if you could climb up to them. I was with Helen and Betty, but Betty felt ill and disappeared below. She was from British Columbia — a tall, friendly person whom I had never met before boarding the ship. We were to become very good friends, in both Sicily and Italy, and would correspond after the war. We had lunch, and then slept, thereby missing P.T. Later we attended a lecture on malaria, which was perfectly terrible! A passing M.O. was heard to say about the lecturer, "She was much worse than the mosquitoes and had quite a velocity!" We then had tea, and Don and Gig, very nice lads from Edmonton and Peace River, sat and talked to us. There was pork for dinner, and later a ship's concert on B Deck, which was very good. We went to bed about 1100 hours, under orders to sleep in our undies!

On Sunday we didn't go to church, but lay on the rafts. At 1130 hours there was some action — depth charges were dropped! All the ships scurried up into the convoy. It was rumoured that a German submarine had been sunk almost beside us. Very exciting! We hurried through lunch, although another depth charge was dropped while we were eating. Afterwards it was all calm, and we lay on the rafts until we were too hot. We had chocolate bars and tea with the five men we met the first day on board. It was announced that we would begin receiving our ration of mepacrine to prevent malaria the following night. We went to bed late, not going below until precisely 2154 hours.

In our cabin there was no place to sit, so we either had to stand, or half-lie on a bunk with our backs to the wall. Water was turned on in the cabins at 6:30 a.m. and we took turns getting up first, as only one person at a time had room to wash and dress for breakfast. One day we were issued a book of bank cheques, or "chits." As officers, everything issued to us would be charged and taken from our bank accounts. We could only write a prescribed number of cheques a month, whether we had the money in our accounts or not. As junior officers it was five cheques a month, for five pounds each. Later, we received one pair of khaki slacks and leather gaiters, the latter to be worn whenever we were aboard a ship.

We were told that when we arrived at our destination we would be living in tents, two to a tent, and that we could choose our tentmate. We were given a very odd lecture, considering the obvious fact that we were headed for the Mediterranean — "The Alaska Highway"!

It was a red herring, meant to make us think we weren't going where we were going.

CHAPTER EIGHT

The Mepacrine Lunch

Although our convoy had passed near Gibraltar we could see nothing, as of course there were no lights anywhere. A naval officer pointed out to us where the island was located. After entering the Mediterranean, we stayed with the convoy — most of which was headed for Sicily to participate in "Operation Husky", the planned invasion of "the underbelly of Europe" — until we were in sight of Algiers, at 4 p.m. on 9 July. The buildings looked very modern and very white in the sun. In the harbour we saw a British submarine and two huge battleships, HMS *King George* and a "sister" ship. We could see No. 5 Canadian General Hospital on board the SS *Franconia*, probably waiting for enough beachhead to be taken in Sicily so they could land safely and set up a hospital. We put down anchor at 5:30 p.m.

At 10:30 p.m. we weighed anchor and went to sea again. While we were in port, the remainder of the convoy had sailed on, and joined an armada of nearly three thousand allied ships and landing craft, ready to launch the invasion of Sicily the next day. Later we learned that fifty-eight Canadian soldiers had drowned earlier, when enemy submarines sank five ships from the front section of our convoy. Five hundred vehicles and many guns were lost. Accompanying us out of the harbour of Algiers were the HMS *Empress of Russia* and a British hospital ship. We watched them through binoculars belonging to some of the officers.

We arrived in the harbour of Philippeville, Algeria, at 5:30 a.m. The *Empress of Russia* anchored just outside the harbour, although the British hospital ship had left. The next day, Sunday, we were still aboard the *Nea Hellas*, and now the *Empress of Russia* had disappeared. It was very hot in the bright sunshine, and the harbour buildings glistened. We had breakfast, and at 9:30 a.m. started to disembark onto large barges, beginning with male officers and newspaper-men. We were taken ashore with the HQ Corps troops. We wore wool suits and full gear, but this time were allowed to take off our heavy backpacks while we waited in the harbour sheds for transport.

At last it was our turn; we picked up our gear and were soon on the dock and loaded into huge lorries. We were told that some American nurses had landed at Bone, further east, and that they had waded ashore! With their kit! So we assumed there was an American hospital in the area. We were told that our hospital site was twenty-five miles inland. We drove through Philippeville, along wide avenues with central boulevards lined with palm trees. There were many Arabs on the streets, male and female, the latter in black cloaks with shawls over their heads, with only their eyes showing.

We were taken first to Canadian Corps Headquarters, a very large holding unit in the midst of a forest of cork trees. We were put down in front of a row of metal Nissen huts (which I learned had been invented during the First World War by Lieutenant Colonel Peter Nissen, a Canadian military engineer), in the same area as the HQ officers and the newspaper reporters.

We were twelve in a hut — not two in a tent as we had been told — but we were allowed to choose our hut mates. I was with, amongst others, Florence, Beth and Bernie. Then we were directed to lunch, but first we had to find our mess tins, enamel cups, knives, forks and spoons to take with us. We decided to take our collapsible canvas stools as well. There were a lot of picnic-style wooden tables, and one great communal kitchen, with the cooking done outdoors. There was a long line of men waiting to be served, so we joined the queue.

The menu consisted of raw onions and sliced tomatoes, bully beef from tins, and hard biscuits. The tea was thick, almost like syrup, with milk and heavily sugared. I hate sugar and milk, but drank it anyway. We had been advised never to drink water, but always tea. You rinsed your mess tin and utensils in a big tub of water — not very hygienic, after hundreds had rinsed theirs in it already.

We were "confined to barracks" for forty-eight hours, and concluded it was because it was an all-male camp — it was certainly for our safety. We were always "CBed" after a move for protection from the locals, and the war. However, we attended church outdoors, a "drum head service" combining different regiments, and afterwards attended a sing-song. The war correspondents came along also. We were still in our navy skirts and shirts.

That first night I slept without a mosquito net. Most of the girls in the other huts were already ill. Everyone called the accompanying vomiting and diarrhoea "Gypy tummy", and we were to have it intermittently in Sicily and Italy as well. We would always have a bottle of sulphaquanadine handy, and just drink it from the bottle. "We must be tougher," I thought.

On 13 July, two days after our arrival, we queued and had breakfast at 8:30, and then went to a staff meeting with the Matron. We were told to take a mepacrine pill during every lunch except Sunday, to prevent malaria. After we settled, there would always be a bottle of mepacrine on each table, and we were responsible for taking it. Eventually, a dye from the mepacrine would give our skin a yellowish tinge, and mine would develop a coppery tint when I got tanned by the sun. But the whites of our eyes did not turn yellow as was the case with hepatitis.

We were delighted to be issued with the tropical kit of the Auxiliary Territorial Service, the British women's army: khaki cotton slacks, skirts, knecktie and a "bush shirt", a kind of tropical jacket which had long sleeves, four pockets, side slits, and buttons up the front. There was no need to wear a shirt under it, and it was quite cool. All officers wore them. The British have always worn such garb in tropical countries, even in the nineteenth century during the years of the Raj. They are still worn in those areas, even though the British are long gone. We removed our insignia — the pips and cloth CANADA badges — and sewed them on our new bush shirts.

Unfortunately, the Matron said we could not wear the khaki uniforms yet. Nor were we allowed to cool off by going swimming at the beach, which was two and a half miles away, as a soldier had recently drowned and they were still searching for his body. He was a victim of the very heavy undertow in this area of the Mediterranean. It was very hot — a hundred degrees — but not humid. And the sand was always blowing around into everything, even our food. The night of the 13th of July we had a windstorm and some rain.

No. 100 British Hospital was near us, located near the shore. There were also Australian and New Zealand hospitals in the area, so that along with the Canadian hospital we represented a good portion of the Commonwealth. The British had lovely blue blankets on the patients' beds, which were all under large marquees, with thirty patients in each. Their patients were allied air force personnel, as well as Germans and Italians, and it was said they had some Canadian casualties. The officers' tents had wooden floors; we never had wooden floors in any of our tents, either in North Africa or Italy — even in winter! And, unlike the officers in No. 100 BH, we washed our own clothes — although nothing was ironed, just wind-dried. The nurses were dressed as we were when we worked, in a blue uniform with white apron, leather belt, and white veil.

We were issued with mosquito nets, and hung them over our beds. The nets had a wooden bar on top which you hooked on the wall above your bed, and then you tucked the netting in all around your sleeping bag — or mattress, if you had one. We had iron beds in the Nissen huts; they had mattresses on which we slept in our sleeping bags.

On 14 July we were issued with an airmail letter form with a three-penny stamp on it, to send to Canada or elsewhere. Our weekly ration. We also got an issue of fifty British cigarettes in a round tin, and two packages of matches. I didn't smoke but decided either to give my cigarettes away or use them for barter. Someone told me the Arabs would exchange fruit, notably melons, for them. One of the

English officers brought me a box of fruit while I was in Algeria — a lovely gift; I gave him soap in return.

We made tea outside the hut in the afternoon, and Betty and I went up and sat on a hill. Swimming was now sanctioned, so some of the nurses walked to the beach, afterwards having the good luck to hitch a ride back in an American ambulance. In fact, there was always one stationed at the swimming place. Some of the officers who had been on board our ship came to visit. Some of them I would see all through the war — no matter where we moved they would come along to our mess, or at least write to us. I had an early supper, went to bed and slept very well.

By 15 July not so many nurses were ill, so we had our pictures taken as a group for publicity purposes. Betty and I walked to the Post Office, where she was handed an airmail letter which had been sent to her from North Africa two months before; it had been to England and had now come back.

I went to an outdoor movie unexpectedly with Helen at the American camp; it was **Babes on Broadway**. The night was lovely and cool. During the movie our hosts served us chicken, grapefruit juice, and a terribly sour red wine; we just poured it on the ground, but it was generous of them to give it to everyone. We came home about 11:30 in a jeep.

Five days after our arrival we had breakfast as usual, and then were told to pack all our gear — suitcases, trunks, large packs — ready to move to a new site at 1400 hours. Things happened all of a sudden in the Army! But we didn't move. Instead, we sat outside the hut for the afternoon. Then we walked down and went swimming. The water was very rough, and, as reported, there was a heavy undertow. I swam out too far and felt the undertow, and it was hard work to get back. I would not go that far ever again. We marched back accompanied by members of the British Dental Corps, who gave us tomatoes and onions, and complimented us on being able to keep up with them.

We said, "We should, as we trained hard in England before we left." As a result of this we were invited to visit No. 100 British Hospital.

The next day, 17 July, we moved by troop carriers to our new camp. It was a very nice place by the sea, near the shore but perched above it, clean and airy. There was a lovely view of the bay. It was going to become a British convalescent hospital, but there was nothing for us to do. However, we were to be here for only a few days. We were in nice tents, with a double fly top — two nurses in each. We had iron beds, mattresses, white sheets and a pillow — with a white pillow case. Luxury! Also showers. Our tents were in rows, of which there were about fifty. We also had a large dining marquee, with long tables and benches, where breakfast would be served at 7 a.m., lunch at noon, and dinner at 7. We could go swimming down below, where the water was warm and calm, and without an undertow. We were at last wearing our khaki tropical clothes, a wonderful change — very cool and smart.

The next morning we were up at 6 a.m. and that day enjoyed two swims. We also prepared for an inspection by General Andrew McNaughton, head of the Canadian Army, which was to occur the following day. General McNaughton turned out to be a tired, elderly man. He welcomed us, and spoke very simply and quite informally. He told us he was very pleased that the 1st Canadian Division was in the Battle of Sicily, although he had not been there himself and had little to tell us. The Canadians were attached to the British 8th Army under Generals Montgomery and Alexander, and as they were not to be a separate Canadian Corps, it was not necessary for General McNaughton to be there. He said he was glad that we were to look after the casualties. Following the inspection, we went to an ENSA concert in the evening at the British Rest Camp not far away. (The "Entertainment National Services Association" provided entertainment for the allied forces.)

On 21 July we heard we were to move again; we would leave for El Arrouch in two days. We would have to be up at 5 a.m. to leave at six.

We were still receiving mail from Canada and England regularly, although our parcels from Canada usually arrived in chaos. That day I received an airmail letter from my mother telling me my father was still very ill. During the night I myself became ill, and had severe chills. By morning I had dysentery.

The next day I was sent to the new site by ambulance, with another nurse who was ill. It was a journey of twenty-four miles. We were given pill opi before leaving, and recovered fairly quickly. We had sulphaquanadine for dysentery, and seemed to be continually taking it. We each had a bottle, and drank from it directly. The pill form of this medication was sent to the troops, as it was easier for them to carry.

Once in Al Arrouch, we found ourselves in a huge encampment, in a large field close to the Atlas Mountains. We were now part of No. 15 Canadian General Hospital, with its 1,000 beds. We helped put up tents and then beds, which we made. Being part of the British forces, we now had the lovely blue blankets seen — and envied — earlier in the British hospital. Our hospital tents were the same as the British marquees, three grouped together to form a ward, with a small area where they were joined to form an office. Each tent held thirty patients, with a side table for each. A separate tent served as an operating room, an x-ray department and a dispensary. Whenever surgery was performed the flap of the operating tent was closed in an effort to maintain a sterile environment. All operations were done early in the morning while it was still relatively cool.

There was a separate compound for male officers, one for nursing sisters, one for NCOs, and one for the ranks, all under canvas, with two in each tent. Each compound had its own mess for relaxing, and also dining, as each had its own cooks. Later, showers and latrines with canvas walls would be built for each compound. There was a large tent for the Orderly Room, small tents for the Colonel's and Matron's offices, a post office, padre's office, and a chapel. Our mail was always put in the mess tent, laid out on several mission-style tables. It was an extensive setup, and all compounds were under guard twenty-four hours a day. Each was surrounded by wire fence with barbed wire on top, with tin cans hanging from it to give the alarm. There was also coiled barbed wire around the whole encampment, which was guarded continually, as the locals were notorious for stealing.

The nursing sisters had a large mess tent which was like a sitting room, very comfortable and full of leather furniture, including huge armchairs like those found in a men's club. How that furniture had arrived was a mystery, and it was very surprising to see it here in all the sand! However, every unit or regiment in the British Army had the same furniture. Large clay urns hung from ropes from the tent poles, full of drinking water mixed with the famous English Rose's Lime Juice, used to disguise the smell and taste of chlorination tablets used to purify the water. The water was cooled by the urns, which were clay and porous, and the shape of those in the Ali Baba fairy stories.

Although we had our own mess, we ate with the medical officers in another marquee, sitting at large wooden tables, five aside on benches. The flies were numerous — and fierce — so the food was covered with fine white netting held down with beads sewn around the edges, as were the jugs and cups. These flies were probably the cause of our enteritis and dysentery; they lit on everything, and we fought them off as we ate. If one's shirt back was damp with sweat, it was at once covered with flies. We each had a "horse-tail" to swish them away.

I was told we would be able to have clear tea soon, instead of a mixture made from a brick, somehow composed of milk, sugar and tea. There was a huge cauldron in which the cooks boiled water, and then threw in the brick. We drank tea all the time, as there was very little pure water. The cooks made hot biscuits and buns for morning ten o'clock tea, and for afternoon tea, and we always carried our own enamel mugs on our belts. We used toothpaste to remove the frequent tea stains from the mugs.

I was working with malarial patients, some of whom died from one type of malaria. We did blood smears to find the special microparasite that causes the disease, which is left in the body from bites by the anopheles mosquito, found in North Africa and other Mediterranean countries, including Sicily and Italy. When the mosquito bites, it injects its "sputum" into the body. A drop of blood was taken from a patient's finger, put between glass slides, and placed under a microscope. This was done when the patient's temperature was high — 103 degrees or more — and during a chill caused by the activity of the parasite. We had to be accurate with the tests; if the diagnosis was positive, the patient was put on medication specific for malaria. Besides, such a diagnosis could also affect the patient's future medical coverage and pension, when he returned to Canada.

By this time, all the Commonwealth hospitals — British, Australian, New Zealand and Canadian — had moved into the same area, so we were one great sea of hospitals. We were friends with the officers attached to the British hospital, and were amused to see them observe their British August 1st Bank Holiday even here!

Funnily enough, we had our first issue of beer at a concert given by ENSA, and although I was not fond of beer, in the heat it quenched one's thirst. We were very surprised to receive a bottle each, and free, as later we always paid for our drinks in the mess, including our ration of a bottle of whisky or gin a month. ENSA also provided small boxes of fruit, which was wonderful, as we had had so very little in England. In Algeria we found the local melons delicious and plentiful, and they were even sold on the beach. We went swimming often, even though we were again a fair distance from the Mediterranean. Miramar, on the coast, was a lovely place to go for the day on swimming parties, and there was a British officers' club there.

It was very hot — well over 100 degrees — which made the wounded patients ill and uncomfortable. They were from Sicily, as were many more soldiers with malaria and hepatitis. There is a wind called "Sirocco", that blows strongly and keeps sand in the air always. We heard that part of the cork forest surrounding Corps Headquarters had caught fire, and the wind fanned the flames. One night a very bad Sirocco forced us to get up and hammer the tent pegs in further, to keep the tents from blowing away. Needless to say, the sand did not hold the pegs well. The canvas tops covering most of the tents were blown away, and a number of the big tents were blown down. Our clothes blew in and around the tents, which was appreciated by the local looters, who were always hanging around the compound looking for anything loose. As the hospital tents had been blown down as well, we had the Army come in the next morning to put up the tents and tidy the place.

We had a day off each week, and always hoped someone would take us on tourist trips to Oran or Constantine. Oran is on the Mediterranean, and had beautiful beaches as well as an American hospital and a British officers' club. Constantine is a very old city in the Atlas Mountains, situated on two mountains connected by a bridge over a great ravine. There was a casino and a British YMCA there. It was in Constantine that I heard of the unconditional surrender of the Italians on 8 September, and of the scuttling of their ships.

When we were out of our unit area we wore our sleeves rolled above the elbows in daytime, with a skirt and no necktie, although we always carried a basket containing our slacks and a tie. At sunset we had to roll down our sleeves, put on a tie, and change the skirt for slacks, as mosquito protection. We changed wherever we could. Although we wore small khaki cotton bandanas over our hair while we worked, we had to wear a khaki beret when we left the unit. However, I still did not have one, and as they were impossible to buy I was always trying to borrow a beret. This was when I was forced to go up and down the lines of nurses' tents to find the proper headgear!

We were still doing our own laundry, drying it on the guy ropes of the tents, and wearing it "wind-blown." We were now sleeping in canvas cots without mattresses, and had collapsible canvas baths, canvas stools which we used as bedside tables, canvas basins on cross wooden legs, and canvas pails for our rations of washing and bathing water. (This was prior to our acquiring showers.) We were billed on our bank accounts for anything issued, such as cots. But all in all, we appeared clean and well turned out. I even kept my skirts and pants between my sleeping bag and my cot to keep a press in them.

Two nurses arrived from No. 5 Canadian General Hospital in Sicily. No one seemed to know why or how they appeared. On 29 August six nursing sisters left on a troopship from Philippeville for Sicily. They were replacements, as nurses were constantly being sent back to England. At this time we had only seventy-eight patients, but forty were admitted in one day. I was on night duty for two weeks, and it was so hot it was very difficult to sleep in a tent in the daytime.

I was invited to a party given by British Army officers from an artillery regiment attached to the American Army. They had a tiny dance floor made from crushed tin cans, and the music was from a calliope, which they claimed had been abandoned by the Americans in battle. The machine to crush the cans was also said to be American. Who was I to doubt their story? The British officers told us they had tried to rescue everything that the Americans left behind, even tanks. They themselves had been told that it was very difficult to replace a tank, but men were expendable! They had then tried to get the abandoned tanks back to their own lines.

On 28 August a cable from my family reached me with news that my father had died on the 16th. I asked the Matron formally for permission to cable my mother, but she said there were many people with deaths in their families, and promptly dismissed me. No sympathy! One of the padres came to me and said he could send a cable for me via the Red Cross. Although I had told no one except the Matron about my loss, he must have learned about it from the Orderly Room or the Post Office. So with his help I cabled my two brothers in England and my family in Canada.

As the Matron had rightly said, "Life goes on."

Part Five — Up to Sicily

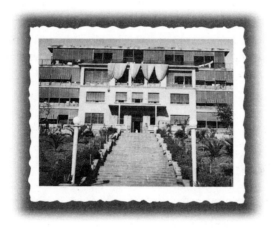

CHAPTER NINE

A Little Wine With Your Spam?

The men of Canada's 1st Infantry Division and 1st Army Tank Brigade, who had formed the bulk of our convoy from England, had gone on to fight in Sicily as part of the British Eighth Army. General Eisenhower, who had commanded the victorious American/British force in northwest Africa, was put in charge of the invasion force, which consisted of the Seventh U.S. Army under General George ("Two-Gun") Patton in the west, and the British Eighth Army (the famed "Desert Rats") under General Montgomery in the east. The Canadians, commanded by Major-General Guy Simonds, performed with great courage and effectiveness. Sicily was in the hands of the allies by 17 August, thirty-eight days after the landing.

A month prior to victory in Sicily, No. 5 Canadian General Hospital had arrived in the harbour of Augusta aboard the SS *Franconia*. Fearing for their safety, the allies had rushed them south to Syracuse, where they had set up shop in a former mental hospital. In the meantime, the *Franconia* had been sunk in Augusta harbour, taking to the bottom all the belongings of the personnel from No. 5 CGH.

In September, five nursing sisters from El Arrouch were required to go to No. 5 CGH, which by this time had moved north from Syracuse to Catania, still on the Sicilian east coast. I was called to the Matron's office and asked if I wanted to transfer to No. 5, as everyone in the small unit I had started with in England was being given this opportunity. I agreed to the move. She said she was sorry to lose me, a compliment I was surprised to get.

While waiting for orders we packed everything, even the cots, but on 30 September we were confined to barracks, so we unpacked everything. We were in limbo — not on No. 15 CGH staff, not on No. 5 —

just in between, waiting to move. We had been struck off strength on No. 15, so didn't work. No one was really in charge of us — we were just five nurses being transferred — so even though we were told not to leave the unit area, we did.

Finally, on 6 October we were told we would leave in the morning, crossing the Mediterranean on a British hospital ship. The ship was to arrive from Sicily, drop off Canadian casualties, and take us back to Sicily, where they would pick up more wounded. So we packed again.

We left El Arrouch by lorry at 8:30 a.m., and were taken to Movement Control for tickets — actually permission to travel. I was issued with "Form AF W3060", an "Embarkation Card" signed by the "Colonel, ADMS Philippeville area." Then we were driven to the harbour and boarded "Hospital Ship AA." We sailed at 10 a.m. on a clean, shining ship — with very good food!

There was actually steak on the menu in the naval officers' wardroom, and when I saw that, I said, "How wonderful, I will have the steak!" The nurse next to me said, "Yes, I will have the steak also." The naval officer across the table looked at us rather oddly and said, "I wouldn't if I were you." Others said the same, but didn't elaborate. When the steak arrived it looked lovely, and we started to eat. Nothing happened — in fact, it was very good. Suddenly the other nurse gave a startled cry, and we looked to see that she had cut into a very large white slug inside the meat! I turned mine over quickly, but it seemed all right. I must have eaten the slugs, in which case they tasted quite good! Great exclamations of, "We told you not to order them!" I am sure the reason they didn't tell us why not was because they thought it would be a great joke to play on the inexperienced and naive Canadian nursing sisters. But we weren't embarrassed. They explained it had been nearly a year since the ship had been refitted and stocked, and it was due for it soon.

Slugs excepted, the meals on board were far better than any we had had in the Army, and everyone was very friendly and kind. After our steak, we were taken into the bar and stood a drink, and made members so that we could then buy our own drinks. Thrifty indeed!

We put into Tunis before going to Sicily, to pick up a new ship's captain to replace the current one, who was going on leave. We were far out in the middle of Tunis harbour from 10 a.m. to 6 p.m. the next day. I was delegated to ask the Matron for the required permission to swim. For some reason she concluded we did not know how, so six sailors were sent with us to make sure we did not drown!

We left Tunis and sailed alone around the island of Pantelleria during the night. Pantelleria had been taken in six days — in January 1943 — by the British, who dropped five thousand tons of explosives on its eastern side. The airstrip there was used as an allied base for the Sicilian campaign. Our whole ship was lit up, with a huge red cross in bright evidence. The next day we saw an Italian hospital ship also sailing by itself — perhaps it was safer that way. We then passed several allied freighters in convoy, heading for North Africa. We were taken on a tour of our hospital ship. Beautifully clean bunks for patients were located one deck below the officers' quarters, along corridors on both sides of the deck. There was also a perfect operating room. The nursing sisters, in blue uniforms with white aprons and veils, were ready to receive casualties. We slept in the officers' ward, in swinging iron cots on stands with moveable sides, the most comfortable way to sleep in a moving ship.

Canadian Corps Headquarters had moved from Algeria to Catania, Sicily. We landed there on the fourth day out, 10 October, were picked up by an ambulance and taken to the hospital, high up on the hillside above the city. The hospital was a five-storey, flat-roofed building at the end of a long winding driveway. It had originally been a tuberculosis sanitorium, one of many built by Mussolini. From the hospital the view over the town and harbour was beautiful, and we could see Mount Etna belching flames, above and north of us. There were no elevators; the Germans had used the building as a hospital before us, and had bedevilled them before retreating. However, a winding circular stairway led up the five flights. We would discover later that when it rained, rivers of water would run down the surrounding mountains, but we were issued with high rubber boots just in time.

We climbed the four flights of circular stairs to the nurses' residence on the fifth floor, a strenuous activity. The dining room and mess were on the roof; the former had wooden tables, and the latter was furnished with leather chairs. We five nurses were given one room with a window on the north end, and we set up our canvas cots and mosquito nets, stowed our trunks — which always just fit under the cots — and were ready to report to the Matron. However, we were told she had been wounded by shrapnel in a German attack, although not seriously, while in the mess, so we reported to her assistant. In fact, just before we arrived twelve nursing sisters had received shrapnel wounds when an anti-aircraft shell fell on the roof at the north end of the building, where our mess was located.

On the evening we arrived, two of us were invited by one of the sisters of No. 5 CGH to accompany her and her American boyfriend, a colonel and the head of a unit, to visit his outfit just outside Catania. Her promise of ice cream was enough to tempt us to go! The Americans were quite different from the British and Canadians, being so much more informal, in both manners and dress. They had an immense ice cream mixer — as large as our concrete ones! — and there was enough delicious ice cream and macaroons, served on china dishes, for the entire unit.

As we were on our way back to Catania, we had just rounded a corner when we suddenly saw in the jeep's headlights two bodies on the sidewalk. We stopped, got out and checked, and discovered they were Canadians, and both were dead. Their boots had already been stolen, even though we had obviously arrived just after they had been killed. An officer stayed with them as we continued to the hospital to get help. It was terrible to think that these two young men had been killed for their boots! And to realize we might have helped them if we had arrived sooner. It made me remember that we were in a war zone, and although this part had been defeated, it could still be very dangerous.

This was not the last time I would encounter tragic deaths of this nature. The Sicilians themselves, travelling around in their beautifully painted caravans pulled by a horse or a donkey, were a menace. And the Mafia was another danger. They probably hated us waging war on their island — bombing their homes, tearing up their fields, crops and orchards. No wonder they stole so much, just trying to live in a terrible war where no one was safe. For me, the essence of my experience in Sicily was the contrast between the rich and the poor, in a society trying its best to cope with horrible living conditions. One could look up at a stately cathedral, and then look down at a child begging for a piece of bread.

I was assigned to a medical ward where all the patients had hepatitis. It is an extremely debilitating disease, and they were miserably ill with nausea and vomiting. Many were on stretchers in the corridors, as well as in beds in a large room. As we had very little medication — or even suitable food — for them, they were sent to a base hospital as soon as possible. At times they were taken by ambulance to the airport, where they sometimes had to wait all day, only to be returned at night. It was either the weather or the enemy, and we had no rations for them. We sent them off again the next morning. They would usually go to No. 15 CGH in El Arrouch, and then on to England.

According to a booklet in the series "The Canadian Army at War", issued by the Ministry of National Defence in 1943, "The total (Canadian) casualties during the Sicilian campaign were 173 officers and 2,261 other ranks", and of these, "38 officers and 447 other ranks were killed or died of wounds." It was generally considered, however, that the number of casualties from hepatitis and malaria was greater than the number wounded in battle.

While we were in Sicily we dressed in khaki, with pieces of cheese cloth or cotton khaki used for veils to tie around our heads, because it was impossible to keep our white starched veils clean and pressed due to lack of water. However, always the head had to be covered! Later we were issued with woolen clothes, because November and December are cold months in Sicily, and the hospital was without heat. Although ours were not, the patients' clothes, boots, belts and equipment were sent to be sterilized, to kill all bugs and germs. Sometimes the leather shrank, requiring replacement clothing.

We were each told to take one of the round tins in which we got our weekly ration of cigarettes and matches, punch holes in the top, and take it to the QM stores to be filled with a pink powder. We were then to dust the seams of our slacks, jackets, shirts, as well as our mosquito nets and canvas cots. We also sprayed the patients' beds, clothing and nets. (When DDT came out on the market after the war, I was sure we had experienced the original, with a number instead of a name.) But still there were lice, bed bugs, and fleas! The fleas were the most persistent; I was sitting at a glass-topped table while on night duty, and watched fleas hop from me onto the surface of the table! It was a losing battle, but everyone was in the same boat, and we didn't seem to suffer any ill effects. However, a year later we would find our hair falling out, and decide it was caused either by the pink powder, or the mepacrine tablets. In fact, today it is known that one of the side effects of taking mepacrine over a prolonged period is loss of hair. There was also a rumour that mepacrine would make us sterile — the girls talked about this often. But if you took your mepacrine, you would not get malaria. For us it was simple, because it was always on the table before us, whereas for the troops mepacrine was a luxury.

In Sicily, and later in Italy, we always had carafes of red and white wine on the table. We never drank water, or had it in drinks. Our diet was Spam, bully beef, bread, and an excellent variety of cheeses. Many of the staff did not like cheese, but I lived on it in Sicily and Italy. It was rumoured that the Canadians had captured a German food dump, as we were fed various types of German cream cheese in toothpaste-like tubes, which I found tasty and nutritious. We had an abundant supply of oranges, a good source of Vitamin C. Often the walking patients would go out with an empty pillowcase, and return with it filled with oranges. I have never eaten such good oranges since. In North Africa we had been given lemons, which we ate like oranges, only with sugar.

In Catania we had our first bath tubs since leaving England, although ironically we had only enough hot water for an occasional bath. Due to the water shortage we had to take "French baths" instead — sponges and talcum powder. We wanted to be clean, and to smell nice! We had so little water that, after a sponge bath, we rung out the water and washed our underwear in it. During cold weather, we then put the water in a hot water bottle, which we placed in our sleeping bag.

The Canadian Army in the Mediterranean was enhanced, preparatory to becoming a full corps, at the end of 1943. Consequently, additional medical units were set up in southern Italy, including three general hospitals and two casualty clearing stations. No. 1 CGS went to Andria near the east coast, No. 3 CGH to Avellino, just east of Naples, and No. 14 CGS to Caserta, north of that city.

No. 14 CGH was almost lost en route to Italy. The evening of 6 November the SS *Santa Elena*, carrying all No. 14 personnel, including one hundred nursing sisters, was attacked by German bombers off the coast of Philippeville. The ship was hit by an aerial torpedo and a bomb, and everyone aboard took to the life boats. Fortunately, they were all picked up by an American destroyer and a troop ship, the SS *Monterey*. To board the latter, they had to climb scramble nets — most difficult, especially in a rolling sea. One nursing sister fell forty feet, but was rescued by a Chinese cook from the *Santa Elena*; he was on a raft when he saw her fall, and dove in to get her. Later, the *Santa Elena* would sink as she was being towed into Phillipeville harbour. The nurses were put ashore and taken to No. 15 CGH at El Arrouch, where the Red Cross proved wonderful, supplying them with cashmere sweaters and cosmetics and whatever else they needed — except uniforms. Later they would obtain the khaki A.T.S. tropical and winter uniforms from the Canadian QM stores in Caserta.

Our social life in Catania was very active, with the presence of the British Eighth Army, including the Canadian 1st Division, Canadian HQ, the Americans and the Air Force! Too many men — too few women. Too many deaths. And the same men kept turning up, if they were still alive. Romantic events were always happening. I never worked on an officers' ward, so only met one or two that way. It is very difficult to go back in your life after so many years, especially to something you really don't want to tell everyone about, and even remember again. It's too personal for this. But someone might say to you, "We seem to get along well together," or "Will you answer if I write?" or "Will you write to me?" Very lonely people — we all were. You saw these friends for short times between battles. Sometimes they were greatly changed by the battles — surprised to find themselves alive. At first I would ask an officer why another officer wasn't with him. He might look at me and say, "He was killed." I learned not to ask. They wanted fun, gaiety, parties.

So meeting someone several times and becoming more than friends may be strange — but not in war. Death was always near for the men; even though you thought it could never happen to them, it did. But there were romantic incidents that were comical to me. In Sicily one of the nursing sisters, a friend, came to me to ask if I would repay a favour I owed her. Jessie had two friends who had a forty-eight hour leave, and she needed one more girl. One was a captain, and the other a major. I pleaded I was too tired, but broke down and agreed to go out with them. She was sure I would like them and enjoy the evening.

They were two tall, handsome men. Part way through the evening they let me into their secret, which had been going on for some time, mostly when the Captain wanted to see Jessie. Both men were privates, and had put up the insignia of captain and major to make it legal for them to be seen courting nursing sisters! Jessie, of course, knew all about it.

One hotbed of social life was academic in nature. Italian language classes were organized at the YMCA, where the wife of an Italian professor from Rome taught every morning. It was a very congenial affair, with all sorts of officers attending. Being able to converse with the local hospital workers, who spoke no English, was extremely productive. One day the teacher came with a great hamper of big grapefruit. She called out the names of those who had enrolled, and gave one to each of us.

As we went further afield, in and around Catania and down the coast, we found evidence of past battles. We saw burnt out tanks and bombed buildings. Everywhere we looked there were signs of the war that had swept over the land: graves beside the roads; crosses made of wood or sticks with helmets hanging from them — German, Canadian, British. I was told that the men of the Canadian Carleton and York Infantry Regiment from New Brunswick were the first to use donkeys as transport over the difficult terrain of rocky hills. This old and famous regiment had a history which stretched back to the Riel Rebellion, during which they marched from New Brunswick to Manitoba in the winter. They were a very brave group of men, and we had many patients from that regiment, and the rest of the 1st Canadian Division. One memorable day we attended a very impressive Memorial Drum Service at Agira, where four hundred and ninety Canadians are buried.

Lung surgery was in its infancy, and we had numerous sucking chest wounds, as well as many injuries from land mines. I was asked to go to a surgical ward where a patient was asking to see me. The man had been wounded in his right arm, which was amputated at the shoulder, an operation performed by his regimental medical officer after a battle. He had heard in his squadron of the Carleton and York, which was from Woodstock, New Brunswick, that there was a nursing sister from his hometown stationed here, and he wanted to see someone from home, even though he didn't know me. He was very young, and still in shock from the loss of his arm, but it was a great comfort for him to talk with someone familiar with his area.

We took rotated turns being Duty Officer for both day and night. It meant staying up until midnight, answering the telephone, running messages, and looking for nurses for the escorts and friends who were calling for them. During the day, in our mess a home sister (a one-pipper sub-lieutenant) poured tea in the afternoon and welcomed all the live-in guests and visiting officers. There was always a very efficient mess sergeant who ran the bar and the mess. The mess sergeant also ran a canteen, where he sold soap, tooth brushes and paste, etc. He made out the mess bills and put out the mail — and he had the last word.

There was also a dietician, with two pips, who supposedly planned our meals and those of the patients. However, with the rations we had, it was difficult. As to the mess cook, it was rumoured he had a book entitled **Twenty Ways to Cook Bully Beef and Spam**.

But it was only a rumour.

CHAPTER TEN

Christmas in Catania — With a Vengeance!

On 8 November 1943, No. 4 and No. 5 Canadian Casualty Clearing Stations arrived in Sicily. No. 4 came to Catania, No. 5 to the badly bombed city of Messina in the northeast, while my hospital, No. 5 CGH, stayed in Catania acting primarily as a large casualty clearing station. The Army decided we would keep patients no longer than a week — sometimes shorter — as we needed the beds for more casualties waiting for care. Any lightly wounded patients stayed with us, and eventually returned to their units.

Still without a khaki beret, I knew I would be needing one soon, so when I heard that an officers' shop had opened in Catania, Mary and I went to see if we could buy one. They had only black berets worn by the Canadian and British Tank Corps, but I decided to get one anyway. The Matron did not like it, but she allowed me to wear it with my khaki uniform. General Montgomery, who visited Catania while I was there, did not object; after all, he himself wore a black beret decorated with three or four badges, and an odd-looking American jacket lined with sheepskin! And the Air Force officers sported silk cravats!

My lovely navy blue top coat was stolen in Sicily — a great loss, as the weather was turning cold and I needed it. I thought I might find a khaki greatcoat to match the rest of my khaki uniforms. Such a coat was worn by the women of the British Auxiliary Territorial Service. I checked at the Quartermaster's Store in our unit, where they had only one — in a small size, but still too large for me. However, it would keep me warm in the meantime. When the Matron saw me in it, she would look as if I was a stranger, and then say, "Oh, it's you!" I was never sure what to think of this, but I wore the coat for the next two years with my navy and khaki uniforms.

We were given a four-day leave after one of our stints on night duty, and I made arrangements through a RAF officer for six of us to spend our leave at the *Grande Albergo Etna* (Grand Hotel Etna), thirty kilometres from the hospital. The hotel had been built before the war by the Germans, and had been a German headquarters — which included a wine cellar filled with cherry brandy! My friend in the Air Force drove us to the hotel, which prided itself on being within an hour's drive of the Mediterranean. The hotel was actually on the slopes of Mount Etna, nearly two thousand feet above sea level. From the Promenade you could look out and actually see the Mediterranean, and at night the stars were so huge and seemed so close I felt I could reach up and touch them. It was a paradise; all the rooms had hot and cold running water, there was central heating, an elegant restaurant, and facilities for skiing and tennis.

The Grand was used as a "leave hotel" for naval officers from Malta, and there were several in residence, as well as two other women officers. Some naval ratings had been brought in by the officers as their batmen, but they were really there to make up a band, and we danced in the evenings. When he learned I was from Canada, and specifically New Brunswick, one naval officer asked if I knew a Canadian Air Force officer named Dibblee, who was from my province and quite famous. It turned out I did know him; he was older than me, and our fathers had been friends. Small world!

One day we nurses climbed Mount Etna, an all-day excursion. We passed "Nelson's Hut" on the way up, a stone building where everyone paused for a rest. When we reached the top and looked over the crater, we couldn't see anything because of the steam and smoke rising from its centre. At night, flames could be seen flaring high. We passed other groups on the way down, but there were no naval officers, because they had neglected to make the climb. They had decided against it — too strenuous! We were each awarded a pin, in the shape of a boot, for climbing Mount Etna.

We worked hard, but we also managed to have a social life. This was reduced when the British Eighth Army infantry returned to England on leave, prior to becoming part of the Second Front in Europe. However, we managed to attend the opening of the Catania Opera House; it was a very cold night, and even the musicians wore coats, scarves and gloves.

On 14 December Mary and I were told to go to Messina the next day, to help at No. 5 Casualty Clearing Station. We would be assigned to look after three special cases. We left a message for anyone who phoned or came to see us: "We will be back for Christmas!" We were not pleased, but set out with all our gear — everything we owned — by special car. It was a lovely staff car, no less, and we travelled with a Canadian brigadier who was also going to Messina.

After we arrived and had lunch at a Canadian transport group, we were sent on to No. 2 British Field Regiment where they gave us accommodation. No. 5 CCS had experienced bad luck; one of the nurses had fractured an arm and another was ill, so they could not look after patients. Mary and I tossed a coin to see who would take night duty; I lost. We had three Canadian patients: one was an officer with diphtheria who was in isolation; one had been stabbed in the abdomen by an irate Italian; and the third had a chest wound. Where we cared for the patients was where we also slept, and it was all part of the British Officers' Quarters.

The place itself was awful, but nicely located down by the sea, and we could see Italy across the water. We went to the Officers' Club only for tea, as we did not know anybody, and we did not like the officers, who were all British Engineers. We were living in parts of their quarters, and although they allowed us to have our meals with them, they really just tolerated us. I didn't blame them, because our presence was a nuisance.

As Christmas drew near we decided to try and get back to our unit in Catania. As I was on night duty, from 7:30 p.m. until 7:30 a.m., I was in a position to look around to see if anybody would help us. I hoped that somebody in the Canadian transport unit would cooperate, so I went to the officer in charge and asked for two ambulances to take us to Catania. It turned out that I knew him from No. 1 CGH, where he had also been in charge of transport. He agreed to let us have the ambulances, and also the drivers, although he wanted discharge papers for them. I then went to the British officer in charge of us and explained I had transport and that we would like to be in Catania for Christmas. He gave us permission; we never did see the Matron of No. 5 CCS. It was a peculiar situation; we saw an M.O. from No. 5 CCS on arrival and got our orders for the patients from him, but it was the British Engineers' O.C. who gave us permission to leave. It was an odd combination of circumstances, one we had never run into before — but we were in the Army! It was all arranged; we would be leaving early on the morning of Christmas Eve.

I still wonder how we managed to do this without going through all the military red tape! We put the officer with diptheria in one ambulance so he would not infect the other two, and Mary went with him. We had whiskey and water in our water bottles to give to the patients to keep them comfortable, and we also gave a drink to the engineering officers before we left after breakfast. Christmas drinks! None for us, however, as we needed clear heads for the journey.

We stopped at a house, a *casa*, with a Canadian Army sign, and I went in to refill our canteens with water. I sat and talked to the men, and told them our story. They laughed and said we had guts to do it. There was a Christmas tree in the front room — not the kind of tree one would have in Canada, not an evergreen, as there were none — but it was trimmed with Christmas cards, which the Salvation Army gave to soldiers to send home. It was sad to see, because the tree was so pathetic, and the soldiers all looked so homesick. But they were happy that we stopped. They usually saw nurses only in the hospital. I felt sorry for them, but we were pleased to be going back to our unit and friends. If we hadn't done our arranging, we would have been in Messina until the British decided we could leave, or our unit remembered to look for us.

When we arrived in Catania, we checked in so that we could admit the patients, and then reported to the Matron that we had returned. I got the strangest feeling that no one seemed to realize we had even been away! Then we went Christmas shopping downtown. It was raining heavily as we left the hospital, with a stream gushing down the hill.

Now that the battle for Sicily was over, it was rumoured that we would evacuate the patients, and our unit would leave Sicily. Another rumour I heard several times was that on at least one occasion in Sicily, Canadian troops had taken no prisoners for one whole day. Rumours were always being repeated, and most of them turned out to be true — except for those we started ourselves, just to see how long and how far they would go before coming full circle! A good way to have fun! At a party a friend started a rumour that I was a Canadian Indian, as my tan had a copper tint from taking mepracrine tablets. The story went the rounds. Later the Matron took several of us to a party, and told us to be sure not to start any rumours that night; obviously the one about me had reached her.

On Christmas Day we were back at work at our hospital. We decorated the ward, and the Colonel had Open House. We went to the Sergeants' Mess and the Privates' Mess for drinks, as one did at Christmas and New Year's. We did the usual things: cooked and served Christmas dinner to the patients, and ate ours on Boxing Day at a formal dinner and party in the Officers' Mess. Passing the port again, and drinking to the King. And then one could smoke.

I received a Christmas card from a soldier I had had as a patient, who was with the Lothians & Border Horse Regiment. It bore the inscription, "A Merry Christmas & A Happy New Year." "1943" was printed in large letters inside a smoke balloon issuing from the gun of a very large tank!

Part Six — Across to Italy

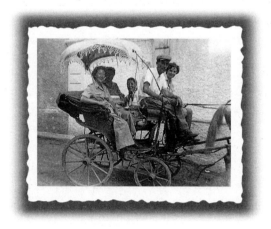

CHAPTER ELEVEN

You'll Love My Mother!

W^e had an air raid in Catania on New Year's Eve 1944, but the hospital suffered no damage. I received a diary from Mary to start the New Year. We cleaned, made beds, and transferred patients to other wards to make room for new admissions. We continued to treat patients, including those who required operations, but were still evacuating them quickly to larger hospitals.

On 8 January, at a cost of three shillings, I attended a dinner dance at the 55 Area Officers' Club, at the *Hotel Villa Politi*, down the coast in Syracuse. Our first Christmas mail arrived on the 15th, and on the 18th the Chief Matron, Colonel Agnes Neill, arrived by plane to inspect the hospital — and us. She was the one who had asked me to join a unit for service outside England. We all liked Aggie Neill; she was generous, friendly, and well able to do her difficult job.

On 12 January No. 5 CCS at Messina went to Italy, ahead of us. Ten days later we were told to pack, and be ready to go to Catania Airfield by 8:30 in the morning. We were to travel by plane to Bari, a port on the Italian east coast, because our hospital was moving too — to Andria, which was near Bari. By this time the Allies had advanced rapidly north through southern Italy, but German resistance was toughening in their determination to keep Rome. As they retreated, the Germans blew up many bridges, and the allied Engineering Corps replaced them with "Bailey bridges" — prefabricated steel panels bolted together — or pontoon bridges, invented by a Canadian officer named Kingsmill (a cousin of my sister's husband), that would even carry tanks. We were allowed one hundred pounds of luggage, and had to jettison the overflow. What a lot of sorting, deciding, and packing! We set aside what we didn't need, and this was sent back to England.

At 9 a.m. six of us, including Mary and Jean, left for the plane with the Matron, as an advance party. We arrived at Catania Airport, but did not have priority clearance to fly to Bari. The Matron and four nurses were allowed to leave at 10 a.m., with a group of high ranking officers, but Jean and I had to wait for another plane, because of our lower military priority. We had tea and sandwiches, and later lunch at the American Transient Officers' Mess at the airport. It was cold, and I was wearing my khaki greatcoat — with two pips up — and Jean was in her navy blue. After many more cups of tea and sandwiches, we were called over the tannoy to board our plane.

We boarded at 1 p.m., and were offered oranges by the British officers, and gum — to prevent air sickness — by the American officers. They said the roughest air trip was across the foot of Italy, across the Gulf of Taranto, because it was always very turbulent. Our luggage was stacked down the centre and we were in small metal backless seats, with our backs to the fuselage and our feet on the luggage, which was in a long pile down the centre. The plane was very warm and the metal seats hot to sit on.

After a smooth flight we arrived at Bari at 4 p.m., and were met by a driver with an ambulance from the hospital. We were hungry, and told him we were going to the American Transient Officers' Mess first. He didn't want to stop, and even said, "I was ordered to return with you at once", but he eventually came in with us under protest, and we all had a very good chicken dinner.

We arrived outside Andria, near the east coast, at 5:30 p.m. Our hospital was under canvas, and was located in a large olive grove in a *sportiva*, a large outdoor sports ground. As usual, our whole area was well guarded. The noise from the many local donkeys — their awful braying — was too much, night and day! When we had first arrived, I didn't know what the sound was, but when I found out I thought it was very funny. The mess was in a house, which provided us with a sitting room, but the nurses were in tents, and ours weren't up yet. We went to have supper in Andria (Another meal! It seems we were always hungry) in another nurses' mess, which I discovered belonged to No. 1 Canadian General Hospital — my original unit! They were in a big building attached to the hospital. I was warmly received, and pleased they were not far from us. After eating, we returned to the olive orchard. We put up our cots in the mess while waiting for our tents to be erected the next day.

There were no floors in the tents, and it was cold enough to freeze water in our canvas pails. We had a small kerosene stove and one lantern. Later, wooden planks were placed between the low wooden cots to keep our feet off the ground, as the mud could be awful, sometimes flowing right through the tents. We wore our khaki clothes in layers; our steel-toed and steel-heeled boots kept our feet very cold. The tents were close together, and you could hear conversations from the others. A tent was not made for privacy, like a room in a house. The latrines were unheated, but they had roofs and walls. Showers would eventually be installed for us, with the benefit of hot water, but the thought of taking a shower in such cold weather meant it would not become a daily event. Neither we nor the patients washed very often. Some of our clothes were sent to be cleaned by the local people, which resulted in several of us having problems. I chanced sending a Viyella dressing gown, but it came back shrunk too small to wear. I had to send to Canada for something washable, and eventually received a red corduroy one that was suitable. It was made by my sister in Halifax, who sent it to me.

We were confined to barracks for forty-eight hours while waiting for our supplies to arrive — beds, blankets, bedside tables, operating equipment, etc. — so we could set up the hospital. However, we could go out with officer friends. The hospital was in large marquees like those we had in North Africa — thirty patients to a tent, three tents to a ward. At the end of the two days, my tent-mate Mary showed up — ill — after a very rough trip. The weather remained very cold, with rain, sleet and wind. We constantly played cribbage, and had playoffs among the nurses, medical officers, NCOs and privates for a prize, a bottle of liquor.

On 28 January an Italian public election was held. We were located in a former Fascist area, Andria being the city where the "Black Shirts" were organized under Mussolini, afterwards spreading all over Italy. Because of the Fascist presence, we were not allowed outside the grounds because of possible danger. They remained very volatile, and could riot at any time.

The first edition of a Canadian newspaper, **The Red Patch,** was issued in February 1944, and we were introduced to "Herbie", a sad-faced cartoon character created by Sgt. "Bing" Coughlin. I saved a cartoon from one issue; titled "Pte. Burp eats at 'Greasy Joe's'", it shows a disgruntled Pte. Burp glaring at his mess tin, while 'Greasy Joe' says to a fellow cook, "Did you hear what he told me to do with the dehydrated cabbage?" The Americans had a paper called **The Stars and Stripes,** and the British equivalent was **The Union Jack,** which had a comic strip called "The Two Types: General Montgomery and General Alexander." They were dressed in odd lambswool jackets, and General Montgomery had a billy can for brewing tea.

We admitted our first patients from the terrible Battle of Ortona on 4 February. Ortona is a medieval town on the Adriatic, directly across from Rome, and it was the site of one of the bloodiest battles of the Italian campaign, with the Canadian troops engaged in house-to-house fighting against fierce resistance. It was difficult for the nurses to comfort the soldiers coming from the battle, sick or wounded, in winter weather with only three kerosene stoves to heat a marquee containing thirty patients. But the men never complained. Their beds were comfortable, with lots of blankets, and we did our best for them under awful conditions.

Again as part of the British Eighth Army, the Canadians had come a long way since crossing the Strait of Messina on 3 September 1943, the day the Italian government surrendered. By this time there were 76,000 Canadian troops in Italy, with total casualties since the invasion of Sicily of 2,110 dead and 9,934 wounded or ill. During February

1944 the Canadians rebuilt their forces, and the First Canadian Corps was formed under Lieutenant-General E.L.M. Burns.

In Andria we nurses ate in an unheated marquee; the tent was so cold we wore wool knitted gloves and coats. To supplement our diets we had our own wooden food boxes in our tents, where we kept eggs, fruit, wine, and other things we could buy in town. We cooked in our mess tins over the little kerosene stoves — if we had enough kerosene, as it was rationed. When we received chocolates in parcels from Canada, they were so stale that we melted them down to make fudge.

While I was on night duty, I wore a suit of men's red ski underwear that had been given to me by a great friend, a Canadian colonel in the Engineers stationed nearby. He accompanied the gift with the words, "Your need is greater than mine." He was going up into battle. They were too big, but I wore them under my khaki slacks, with my own woolies under them, plus a wool khaki man's shirt and pullover, as well as my wool battle jacket and top coat. The ski underwear made the rounds, because when my shift was over I gave them to a friend to wear on hers, and she did the same.

This same colonel had suffered a terrible tragedy. Some of his officers had placed a tin of gasoline, thinking it was water, close to the stove in their tent. During the evening, while they were playing cards, the stove exploded, and two of the men, covered in flames, had run screaming into the night. After the fire was extinguished, it was discovered that three officers had died as a result of the incident.

It was eerie when we were alone on night duty, as no one was ever seen after midnight. One night when I was on duty I received a call on the field telephone from the Orderly Room, telling me an ambulance driver was wanting to see me. When he came to the hospital he had asked if I was from the Royal Victoria Hospital in Montreal, as he had heard there was a RVH graduate at No. 5 CGH. I remembered him from nights on duty in the delivery room (called the "case room") at the RVH Maternity Building. We had to deliver babies in some mothers' homes, and he usually drove us — a McGill University medical student, a nurse from the case room, and at times myself — and waited until we were ready to return. The driver would never leave the nurse alone in a house with the intern, even with the family present. Formerly, he had been an "Al Capone man" in Montreal, and had been shot. He was taken to the Royal Victoria Hospital, and upon recovery expressed a wish to work at the hospital. He became a driver. I would never have believed it if anyone had told me I would one day see him in Italy, but I enjoyed our meeting.

The only times we were warm were when we went with friends who were officers — and had transport — to a restaurant in a hotel in Bari, or to the British Officers' Club five miles distant. At this club women were not allowed in the bar, so we sat in an anteroom and had our drinks brought to us. Here we played a joke on the British officers. Mary had received her Canada Medal with clasp for volunteering, and we told them she had received the Canadian V.C., "for duty beyond daily work." They all believed it, and bought us drinks, but a Canadian officer came in and gave us away, and we had to break down and tell the truth. We actually called it "The Spam Medal"; everybody had one in the Canadian Armed Forces, because we were all volunteers, and it was said that it came along with the Spam! I was overdue in receiving mine, due to my several transfers to various units. However, shortly thereafter we were all wearing our Spam Medals!

Twenty-five Italian guards with rifles, as well as our own guards, were on hand for our protection, because the locals were always hanging around looking for something to steal. I was in Bari one day when I saw bags of flour stamped "Gift of U.S.A." being unloaded from a ship, to be distributed to the Italian people. As I watched, the bags were opened and dumped on the dock, mostly by small boys, who quickly disappeared with their booty.

On a cliff overlooking the ocean at nearby Trani was Neill House — commonly called "Jo's Place", after the home sister who was in charge. Established 1 March 1944, it consisted of a main house and four outlying buildings. It was a nursing sisters' rest villa, containing forty-five beds, where we could go for a day or overnight — for five lire. Only a twenty minute drive away, we got there either by hitch-hiking or a lift from a friend. We could always enjoy a hot bath in a real tub, which was the the most attractive thing about the place! The food was excellent, especially the spaghetti and *zambione al fuora* — and the breakfasts in bed. There was a private beach five minutes away, from which we left for picnics and sailing parties in Trani Harbour. During one picnic I received a marriage proposal from an American officer with a broad western accent, who said, "You'll love my mother!" I hardly knew him, and we all thought it was a joke, but it wasn't!

We were enthusiastic tourists whenever we had time, although we could not have gone far without male officer escorts. One night we all went out in a fishing boat with Italian fishermen. The fleet sailed together, with long lights shining from the prows to attract the fish, which were caught in circular nets thrown out by the fishermen. Another entertainment we attended was a "tin hat" concert, given by a British touring troupe, which was held outdoors in the *sportiva* on a large platform stage. It was enjoyed by all staff and up-patients from No. 1 and No. 5 CGHs.

Mid-March was very rainy, with mud everywhere, necessitating our wearing rubber boots. As a need arose for such things, they would be issued to us. The mud in our tents surrounded the wooden planks. The end of March brought wind, snow and hail. The water froze in our canvas pails, and it was much too cold to take showers. March also brought a new commanding officer, so we cleaned and tidied every-thing in our tents and the hospital in preparation for a very thorough inspection.

On 9 April we attended an Easter Service in Andria, for Canadian troops of the "Central Mediterranean Forces Italy." Although it was a traditional service, the Chaplain asked that we "pray for the King's Majesty, for ourselves, our Cause, our fallen comrades": "Bless our sovereign Lord King George, prosper his forces and those of his allies; decide the issue of this war according to righteousness; have mercy on the wounded; succour the dying; comfort the bereaved; cheer the anxious, uphold the faith of Thy servants and give peace and lasting concord." Although this was a little ambiguous as to who were the good guys and who the bad, the postscript to the "Order of Divine Service" was not: "The Protestant Chaplains of Canadian Troops wish all ranks a Happy Easter, and pray that the meaning of this day of our Lord's sacred triumph may inspire all through struggle and suffering to victory over our enemies." We were always praying for "Victory", and sang "Onward Christian Soldiers." The padres had little portable organs for us to sing along to. Each padre also had a silver goblet, from which we sipped wine during the communion services. We were constantly having our morale boosted. We didn't have Churchill to do that for us, so the padres did it, even at communion.

April 1944 was the heaviest operational period on the Adriatic, and I once stood and watched from Neill House on a very clear day as hundreds of paratroopers were being dropped across the Adriatic Sea. Someone suggested that Greece was their objective, but we never found out.

Our last patients were admitted 26 April. Evacuation started the next day; we were on the move again. On 1 May, No. 1 CGH in Andria also moved. Our Matron was leaving for England, and we awaited a replacement.

We set ourselves up in the marquees which housed the patients, and we were back to using our mess tins and lining up at the outdoor kitchen for meals. Breakfast consisted of fried bread (if there was any), stringy bits of canned bacon, and powdered eggs.

CHAPTER TWELVE

The Red (Light District) and the Blue (Grotto)

W e left at 2 p.m. Sunday 6 May, headed for western Italy. We had been ready since 9 a.m., and spent our time playing cards and singing, "Waiting, waiting, waiting, always bloody well waiting." We were driven in full kit from Andria north to Barletta on the Adriatic coast, where we boarded an ambulance train to cross Italy. Our destination was Caserta, near Naples. We pulled out the seats and made beds, and slept in our clothes, along with the bed bugs and the fleas!

We arrived in Caserta at 6 a.m. next morning, and had hardboiled eggs and coffee for breakfast, thankful it was not bully beef or Spam, or even pilchards in tomato sauce. It was very hot, but we left the train in full pack, wearing our wool khaki clothes. We climbed onto troop carriers, long open transports with benches down each side and two rows in the centre. We sat facing the sides of the vehicle, never to the front or back. We rode about ten miles along a narrow dusty road to Cancello, a very small, poor village.

Cancello was like Algeria — dusty and dirty — and we were covered with grime most of the time. Again we were under canvas, in a stubbly wheat field with the grain growing through the floorboards in the tents, which were very close together. We set up our canvas cots and mosquito nets. We queued for meals, and, as usual, got the main course and dessert together in our mess tins. The latrine, with six seats, had canvas walls but no roof. For washing, there was a long pipe, with holes through which water of a deep rust colour dripped into a long wooden trough. We could take water to our tents to have a bath or wash our clothes, which we dried on ropes tied from the guy ropes between the tents.

We found ourselves in the midst of a large complex, with English, Australian, and New Zealand hospitals, as well as our own No. 5 CGH, all under canvas. There was a sea of tents covering a large area among a few trees, near a very old-looking village on a hill. The narrow and dusty dirt road, not far from us, was heavily travelled at all times by small and large army vehicles. We were once more close to a volcano — Mount Vesuvius, which was quiet at the time, but had been very active. All flying in the area was cancelled while Vesuvius was erupting, because the lava dust was so thick and high in the air, it was sucked in by the engines. Naples was a forty-five minute drive to the southwest, and we were thirty-five miles southeast of Capua, called "Ammunition Hill", located just twelve miles south of the front lines.

Campobasso was a city northeast of us; it was an amazing place, with a huge recreation centre for Canadian troops, with canteens run by the YMCA, the Canadian Legion, and the Knights of Columbus. There were clubs for officers and other ranks, theatres, cinemas, and mobile baths. It was called "Maple Leaf City", and there would be four thousand officers and men there on forty-eight hour leaves at any one time. I went there only once, to attend a big celebration put on by the Salvation Army. After the war, many Italians would emigrate to Canada from this area.

We were waiting again for the hospital marquees and beds to arrive. Since we couldn't take in patients, the hospital organized a bus trip for us to Naples and Pompeii. It was a great surprise to be told a trip was planned, and we were all very excited at getting to Pompeii. The Matron went with us to be in charge.

There were a great many officers and other ranks from the allied armies and air forces at Pompeii, so we were crowded as we walked down its main street. All the sightseers were from the military, either on leave or waiting to go into battle, but it hardly seemed we were in the midst of a war; we were all just tourists! Visiting Pompeii was like going far back into the past, seeing history alive. The main street was made of large blocks of black hardened lava — the original road. But as the guide told us, there was a very old smaller city underneath, that had also been destroyed by Mount Vesuvius, which was less than a mile away. All the major streets were of smooth black lava, and quite wide, with ruts on either side where chariot wheels had worn the stones down. Between the buildings were narrow foot paths.

We went inside some of the houses and found lovely murals on the walls, still in bright colours, and mosaic designs on the floors. There were some tables and chairs, and there were loaves of bread (hardened by lava) and bottles on the tables, and plates and cups. One house had a glass case on either side of the entrance, containing phallic items. Everyone was crowded around to look in the cases! The guide told us they had been put there to signify "a house of ill repute" in Pompeii's "red-light district." In the midst of all this, a hand suddenly appeared on my shoulder. Turning around, I discovered the Matron. I didn't know she was walking behind me. She said, "Sister Carter, you are not wearing stockings! It's against all the rules! Don't let me see it again."

I said, "I'm sorry, but it is so hot!" In fact, I had a good tan, and purposely didn't wear stockings — not telling anyone and never expecting Matron would be near enough to me to be able to tell the difference! Everyone who heard was trying not to laugh at me — strangers as well.

We went from Pompeii to a school, a very large square building, where cameo carving was taught. The cameos were usually oval, and showed a beautiful woman's head and shoulders — a miniature carved from coral, ivory, or semi-precious stone. We visited a large work room where young men at benches created these superb miniatures by hand. There were many for sale, but all very expensive, being set in gold or silver.

By 15 May our new matron had arrived, and we were all set up and admitting patients. We first used penicillin at Cancello, although it was in very short supply. When injected into the patient's badly injured knees and shoulders, it was indeed very painful. There were no penicillin pills — just liquid. Again sickness was a more serious medical problem than casualties, which were admitted directly from the front lines.

During April and May the British Eighth Army had moved from eastern to western Italy to assist the Fifth U.S. Army and the British First Army in the assault on Rome. Atop a mountain at Cassino was a Benedictine monastery, the last key position on the road to Rome. The Canadians had reentered the fighting, and were heavily involved in the Battle of Monte Cassino. They were less than fifty miles from our hospital.

At Cancello I was in the same group of nurses as in Andria, and again I pulled night duty. It was almost impossible to sleep in our tents during the day, even with the flaps open and sides rolled up. It was too hot — a very sudden change from the cold weather in Andria. So we had to find our cotton khaki clothes. In addition, there was heavy traffic on the road beside us, and nursing sisters were leaving for England and new ones arriving continually. However, the old core of nurses remained, even though we were seeing new faces all the time. When on night duty, we would sleep a few hours in the morning and then get up and get dressed.

Sometimes we would go out to the road and hitchhike, carrying our haversacks, tin hats, and gas masks. We also took bathing suits and some money. Sometimes we would be picked up by our own transport, but on our first trip we were given a ride by an English officer and his driver in a halfton truck. Although we had wanted to go to Sorrento, where there was a British leave hotel, the officer took us first to see San Sebastiano, just twenty-five miles from our hospital, where lava from Vesuvius had almost covered the village, leaving the roofs of the houses just visible. The lava under our feet actually burned through our shoes. We never learned how many had been killed, but it was not the first time it had happened to that place.

The scenic drive down the coast road to Sorrento provided a lovely view of Naples, and the Isle of Capri. On 26 May we went to Naples by bus, to a club called "Maple Leaf Gardens", where we had ice cream. The armies had been through this area, and left their signs: "Winnipeg Road", "Buffalo", "Victoria Bridge." In Sorrento, all the good hotels were down by the water, including the place where we stayed, the YMCA Club.

We also managed — finally — to get to the Isle of Capri for a couple of days, and to the Blue Grotto. We had been packed to move yet again but had still not been to Capri. It was difficult to find out how to get there. Finally, on Friday 8 June we got up early, had breakfast, and hitchhiked to Sorrento. Five nurses, with enough gear for a two-night stay at the YWCA Club, we thought at first we should split up in order to hitchhike. But we decided to go all together. Traffic was heavy, so we caught a ride quickly. At the YWCA we had dinner with officer friends who were staying there. Afterwards, they took us to a RAF party at Cocunele, where we were told to take the American launch to Capri.

On 9 June we were up early and caught the launch. It was a forty-five minute trip, and took us around the island to the harbour. There we boarded small boats — two or three to a boat — which took us to the Blue Grotto. At the entrance we had to bend away over, as the opening was so low. It was beautiful inside, seeming like a serpentine. From the moment you entered, everything was blue, including the air itself. The walls were a dazzling blue, and were reflected in the water. I concluded there must be holes in the ceiling to allow light to enter.

When we left the Grotto we returned to the harbour dock and took the *Ferrovia Funicolare* up the high rocky side of the island to Upper Capri. I still have my ticket; it cost me 1.40 lire for a *Classe Terza Discesa*. We were "picked up" by some Canadian officers, who took us to lunch and then to Ana Capri, and around the island. We saw all the expensive shops and the lovely elaborate *casas* of the movie stars, although living conditions for the ordinary citizens were terrible. We caught the funicular down to the dock, but as we were descending we saw the U.S. launch leaving the harbour. We were too late! But when we arrived at the dock the crew of an RAF launch offered to take us back to Sorrento. We returned to the YWCA, from which we descended 435 steps to the shore for a swim.

At Cancello we were able to get new cotton drill slacks from the QM stores to replace our badly worn ones. To make moving easier, we were advised to send some of our clothes to "Surplus Kit" in England, as we had done before we left England by convoy. It was a marvel to me how our belongings were never lost, even though ships were being torpedoed.

One day eight of us were ordered to attend an overnight party — we called such affairs "Command Performances." Although some nurses volunteered for these functions, I never did. This time the Americans had asked for Canadian nursing sisters to attend a party, which surprised us since they had plenty of their own in Italy. The Matron ordered me to put my name on the list. We were to go to Foggia, sixty miles east, for a performance by Marlene Dietrich near the American front line. Everyone knew about Foggia, as the Americans had a radio station there, and their opening line, usually in a southern drawl, was always, "This is downtown Foggia."

Transport was sent for us and we were taken to a Nissen hut where we were to sleep. The next day two jeeps were to drive us to the front line to see the show. Somehow our driver got lost, and we arrived at a crossroads, right in the midst of bombing and strafing! The soldiers on point duty in the American Sector shouted at us in no uncertain language to get out — and fast! So we beat a hasty retreat. The roads were very good in what seemed to be a valley, with very high walls of earth. There were signs at the crossroads, which gave directions to American cities, and the number of miles. We got back to Foggia, but never did see Marlene Dietrich. The next day we were safely back with our own unit. I vowed that that would be the last "Command Performance" I would attend. But I was wrong.

I was invited by a friend in the U.S. Air Force to a dance at American Army Headquarters in Naples. I went, primarily because of the promised food: chicken, ice cream, and chocolate cake! But I also thought it would be a pleasant affair, as there would be an orchestra and dancing. I went in my cotton khaki belted skirt and shirt. Neither had been ironed, but I slept on the skirt the night before and it looked good enough. I wore a khaki necktie and my sleeves were down, buttoned at the wrist against the mosquitoes (as in Orders). I wore a small khaki scarf on my head to keep the dust out of my hair while riding in the jeep. When we arrived at the dance, I went to the dressing room off the front entrance to remove my scarf and comb my hair, while my friend waited in the foyer. I had little make-up, and I didn't even have my purse. I had a silver powder compact, and my only watch — a pocket watch — which both fit into my shirt pocket. In the dressing room I discovered American and Italian women wearing lovely evening gowns, something my friend had deliberately avoided telling me, although I should have expected. They looked at me as though I had no right to be there, and I left the room quickly.

The house was on a terrace which overlooked the Bay of Naples, and there we danced. A British liaison officer to the Americans and I were the only ones in uniform. An American general asked me to dance, and complimented me, as a representative of all Canadian nursing sisters, for being able to enjoy myself in my khaki clothes, when all the other women were in evening gowns. He told me that he and two officers with him had not brought dates, in order to ensure that I would have "a good time." I replied that I had come for the food, which was wonderful! He laughed and agreed, knowing about our rations. The officer I was with usually flew a route from Italy to Russia to England and back, but he was lost on his next flight. After that I received no more gifts of Coca Cola or orange juice, until I was in Rome.

Some friends took us to the "Orange Grove", an outside club in Naples that had a dance floor. Our friends frequently had their jeeps stolen while they were there, and then had to find transport to take us back to our units. One night at the Orange Grove someone accidentally dropped cigarette ash down the back of my khaki battle jacket hanging over my chair, burning a hole. Much to my surprise, back at my unit a few days later I received a Size 1 men's battle jacket, delivered to me by hand. I never learned who had sent it, but I thanked the driver and sent a message of thanks to the anonymous donor. I needed it very badly, and had it cut to fit by the unit tailor.

A team of two medical officers and two nursing sisters left our unit for the front, as a medical team. Two other nursing sisters went to No. 3 British Hospital, which needed more help. More and more casualties were being admitted, and we were very busy all the time. Patients were quickly evacuated to large hospitals, especially No. 15 CGH in Africa and convalescent depots in Italy, including Campobasso.

Some news was always posted on our bulletin board in Part One or Part Two Orders, and we had other news by letter, or from friends whose units were near Naples after being pulled out of the fighting. On 4 June we learned that the Canadian Corps, along with the Americans and the British, were in the suburbs of Rome.

On 6 June we had news that the Second Front in western Europe had begun. That was the official information on our bulletin board, and we read it avidly. Eleven thousand planes, three thousand large ships and many smaller ones, were in the English Channel. Three ports were being invaded, on a front one hundred miles long, and para- troopers and supplies were landing behind enemy lines. Fourteen thousand Canadians were attacking front and centre, as part of the British Second Army, and many of our "Desert Rat" friends in the Scottish regiments of the famous 51st Highland Division were part of it, the ones we had seen the King review in Dorking, England, the ones General Montgomery had taken with him to the African desert and then to Sicily. Surely all of this would shorten — or end — the war!

The taking of Rome was rather overshadowed by this stirring event. However, the Italian campaign had done good service, helping the cross-Channel operation against Normandy by engaging the elite German forces in Italy — and holding them there.

Part Seven — Rome

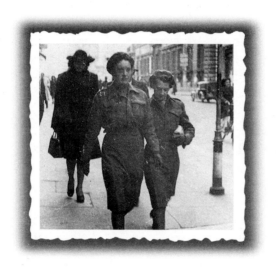

CHAPTER THIRTEEN

I Invade Rome

The fall of Rome was celebrated, and we listened to a speech by King George VI on the occasion. Canada had lost many of its best and most experienced soldiers in Sicily and Italy to death, injury, and illness. Many officers, both senior and junior, returned to England at this time, some of my comrades and dear friends among them, to take part in the Second Front.

We were once more on the move, and everything on the tent wards was packed. Our Colonel went to Rome on 12 June to locate living quarters for us that were as close as possible to where our hospital would be. On 17 June we were up at 4 a.m. and aboard troop carriers by 6 a.m. I was in one of the two centre rows. Constantly moving sideways was not a comfortable way to travel, and not one I would wish to encounter again.

It was an awesomely rugged trip. We went through Monte Cassino, all in complete ruins, burned black. The stench of burning flesh and death was worse than it had ever been in Sicily. Added to that was the smell of burning wood, and another odour which was unidentifiable, but nauseous. We passed a billboard-sized sign with the words, "New Zealand Troops Destroyed by Pinpoint American Bombing." We had often heard and joked about "pinpoint" bombing by the U.S. as they were notorious for missing their targets.

We stopped to eat the sandwiches we had made the day before, and to relieve ourselves behind bushes. We stopped several times just to "brew up." For those who wanted tea, the driver poured gasoline on the ground, put a billy can of water on top, and lit the gasoline. When the water boiled he would put in the tea, sugar and milk. I was glad to have my tea, and had my enamel cup at the ready, packed with my gas mask. We all had our enamel cups with us; I had carried mine everywhere since Algeria.

The drivers were English, and were very good to us. They told us we were the first non-combat convoy headed for Rome since its fall and the declaration that it was an "open city." We drove through small, poverty-stricken villages. We saw a donkey being hoisted by a rope to the second floor of a stone house; it was getting dark and the owners didn't want it stolen. That donkey was the only animal we saw the whole trip; not even chickens! If they had not already been killed, the soldiers would claim to have "liberated" them.

We were tired, dirty, and half-ill when we arrived in Rome at 4 p.m. that evening. There was no real damage; I heard Rome had been hit only once. After travelling through a very poor part of the city, we arrived at a two-storey building. It was a former private girls' school, which had been allotted to us as the Nursing Sisters' Home and Mess.

We were right on the Tiber, across the river from the *Collegio Militare*, the former Fascist Officers' Military Academy, situated on the *Via della Lungara*. The ex-King of Italy's son Albert had trained there. It was now the site of our hospital, and the medical officers and all other staff had already arrived. The building had three stories, and was four-sided around a large courtyard which had been used as a drill ground. An archway served as an entrance into the courtyard. Beside the hospital was the Rome jail, and not far away was Vatican City.

We were a ten-minute walk across a bridge from the hospital. The Tiber was brown and dirty and low, and everything seemed to be floating in it, including the bodies of animals — and human beings. The lights were to be left on in our building all night. I hoped we would not be there long. However, there was running cold and hot water, which was wonderful after only cold water in Cancello.

Eventually our kits would arrive in lorries, and be taken into the school. We were to set up our cots in a large classroom or gymnasium, sixty in the room. My kit would be among the last, and I would end up in a spot in the centre. The process whereby this happened began after we had had dinner and were still waiting for our gear. I was called and told that someone outside was asking for me. It was very dark, and there were three Canadian officers, only one of whom I knew. We had first met on a blind date in Catania, and he was the generous supplier of my red underwear in Andria. The other two had come along hoping to pick up nurses. I couldn't understand how they knew we were coming to Rome, and how to find us. They just said, "Rumours." My friend wanted me to go out with them. I was truly tired after the awful trip, and I hadn't eaten much dinner. I also had to wait for my gear, and put up my cot. He waved it all aside, and said, "Someone will do it for you, I'm sure." So I went out for cognac to pick me up — to brace me.

I was taken to an almost deserted off-limits beer bistro in the basement of a building, with big beer barrels for tables, and chairs made from smaller ones. Three Royal Air Force pilots who had been shot down were there. They had sought sanctuary in the Vatican, but had been deemed prisoners of war, and had just been released after the fall of Rome. They were very thin and looked ill, having had little to eat during their imprisonment. They were glad to be free, and were on their way to find a RAF headquarters.

I returned to the residence to find everyone in bed, with the lights on, and my cot and sleeping bag carefully laid out in the middle of the room. No one ever said who had done the great kindness, although it was also a joke, as there was hardly enough room for me to walk in and out; I had to climb over everyone and sometimes fall while trying to reach my spot. That night I crept over the beds, hardly undressed, and tried to sleep. Not feeling well, I wanted to get up and turn the lights off. The next morning I felt better, but still tired.

My friend from the previous evening came over alone, and we went out to see Rome. Rome was a lovely city — so much history and so many ancient buildings — or parts of buildings. He was a very knowledgeable person, who, from Sicily to Rome, had given me the history of every significant place, and taken me there. There were streetcars running, which gave access to many famous statues and the major ruins, which were in the centre of the city. We found Rome full of troops: American, British, and Canadian. The Roman women were well-dressed. There were no birds or cats or dogs — they had all been eaten. In the Mediterranean area — as in the Far East — people caught birds in nets to eat, both bones and flesh — a delicacy.

That same day we were told we were in the school only temporarily, because the Americans wanted it. They held the government of Rome, and when we first arrived we were under a curfew organized by the Americans. We had to be indoors by 10 p.m. This was later extended to eleven, and then midnight before we left. We were each issued a small card by the Americans, allowing us to live in Rome and run the hospital. It contained our name, rank, nationality, and the name of the hospital. We were to carry the card permanently, as it could be demanded at any time by the American military police, of which there were many throughout the city. The police often asked for the card, more to embarrass us than to check our right to be there. We were allowed to go wherever we liked, but not alone; we were to travel in groups of two or more, at the beginning always accompanied by a male officer.

Rome was a leave centre for all the troops in Italy, and everyone we knew would eventually arrive, either at our mess or our hospital. Anyone on leave had to have, in addition to the identification card, a leave pass. I knew Canadian officers and other ranks who had been arrested for not having one of them, and then held in the American jail overnight — much to their chagrin. One of my officer friends was picked up with his jeep and driver in Rome, and spent the night in the jail in the basement of "The Wedding Cake." This was the name we applied to the magnificent building in the centre of Rome, from the balcony of which Mussolini had delivered speeches. It was the King Vittorio Emanuele Monument and the Tomb of the Unknown Soldier, but now served as American Headquarters. This officer had had his leave pass with him, but not the one needed to live in Rome. He was allowed out the next morning before lunch, very angry!

We would be moving in a few days to another girls' school further up the Tiber, close to the San Angelo Bridge and across from the round *Castel San Angelo*. So we began packing again. In the meantime, we were free while we waited for the hospital equipment to arrive. A concert was held for American troops at the Royal Opera House, under the auspices of the U.S. Army Special Service Division, and tickets had been left at our hospital for anyone who wanted to go. Some of us went and saw **This is the Army,** a wonderful "All-Soldier Musical Show" written by Irving Berlin. Men played all the parts, including "Canteen Hostesses" and "Ballerinas." Imagine our surprise to see Irving Berlin himself, dressed in World War One uniform, conducting and singing his own songs throughout the show! He was a very small, elderly man, and was received with great enthusiasm. He even sang a solo of "Oh, How I Hate to Get Up in the Morning", written when he was a soldier in the First World War. Included in the show was "The Fifth Army's Where My Heart Is", which was printed in the program, and included some timely lines:

> We landed in Salerno, and kept right on the go.
> As we fought our way through Napoli, into Anzio.
> Mile by mile we've been soldiering
> The hard way it seems,
> On the road leading to Rome.
> And without a single doubt
> There'll be things to shout about
> When the Fifth Army comes home.

I wrote beside these lines in my program, "Just not American boasting."

On 22 June I attended a Gala Concert sponsored by "British Army Education for All Allied Forces", again at the Royal Opera House. An orchestra and chorus presented a program of Italian music by Verdi, Puccini and Rossini, and performed by famous Italian opera stars such as Tito Gobbi and Maria Caniglia.

At this time we were eating dehydrated ground meat, cauliflower and potatoes. This was put on your plate dry, with no sauce, and had no flavour. I ate cheese instead, until our cook traded the Italians some Spam and bully beef for spaghetti and tomato sauce. It was a wonderful feast! He said he got the recipe from a Swiss Guard at the Vatican, but used his mother's recipe for the pasta. The meat in it was Spam.

We had a Canadian officers' club in a nice hotel in the centre of Rome nicknamed, appropriately, the "Chateau Laurier", just down a street from the railway station and close to the Forum. The British equivalent was the Crusaders' Club, as well as the Hotel Eden Restaurant in the Borghese Gardens, which was operated by the British NAFFI. An American club was located in The Excelsior, an Italian hotel and the best hotel in town. Other Canadian ranks had Canada Club, in a huge building that was beautifully decorated and had everything anyone could wish for. It looked as though it had been an art gallery.

In fact, I attended an exhibition at Canada Club entitled "Canadian War Art", which featured seventy-six works, mainly watercolours, by Captain Lawren Harris and Major Charles Comfort. The men were described in the brochure as "Official War Artists of 1 Canadian Field Historical Section", and the works as "essentially field sketches, made for the purpose of creating a graphic record on the spot." The painters were praised for having lived under the same conditions as the rest of the soldiers, including making their sketches "under fire."

We enjoyed being tourists for a few days until we started admitting patients. As soon as our supplies arrived, the hospital was set up in the elite military college. Our medical officers were billeted on the ground floor on one side, with other ranks near the back, the Orderly

Room at the front, and the kitchen on the fourth side. Patients were on the second and third floors, which the Germans had used for officers' classrooms and dormitories. When cleaned and set up, the building made a good hospital, which included a laboratory, dispensary, and offices.

We had no electricity at the beginning of our stay, and had to use lanterns after dark. For this reason most surgery was carried out during daylight hours, but if an emergency operation had to be performed the surgeons worked under the light of kerosene lanterns. I had been given two small lanterns in Andria, which were easy to carry around, and I was glad to have brought them on my last move. Later we had electricity sporadically, but it was never very bright.

There had been heavy casualties in the taking of Rome. I was on a medical ward, again with hepatitus and malarial patients. The Germans had opened the dykes and flooded the farmlands, so there were lots of mosquitoes with the resultant increase in malaria; one of our nurses even came down with it. The Allied Army was rebuilding the dykes, and DDT was being used on all ponds and wetlands to stop the mosquitoes from multiplying.

We moved our billet to the next private girls' school, and were now a fifteen minute walk from the hospital. We would cross the San Angelo Bridge, walk by the San Angelo Castle on the right, turn left past St. Peter's Basilica and the Vatican on the west side of the Tiber, and then on to the hospital in "The Academy." It seems we were allowed to use the building as our residence because the Americans did not want it. It had been a school for young girls — that is, judging from the small square sunken baths and the height of the wash basins and toilets! There were about twenty-five of the little baths in a large room, with walkways between the rows for supervision of the students. There was plenty of cold water, and there was hot water too, but it always ran out later in the day. We hardly drank any of the vile tasting water — we had wine, red and white, on the dining room tables, as well as tea and a sort of coffee. The mepacrine bottle was always there, still to be used every day except Sunday.

Our new home was a large square building with a flat roof. The place was old and dilapidated, and even shabbier and dirtier than the previous school, so we had plenty of cleaning to do. We had also cleaned our hospital, but there had been orderlies to help. The only times we didn't clean when we moved were when we were under canvas. We had been told that there always had to be at least one hospital under canvas, for propaganda purposes, so the newsreels could show how we served Canada! There were actually two — No. 15 in Algeria was a base hospital throughout the Sicilian and Italian campaigns, and No. 5 was under canvas twice. Both had endured hard living conditions, although we had done very well in the face of them: the weather, the mud, the food, and the scarcity of water.

We again moved our beds into classrooms, but with only four in each. I was on the second floor, and had only one room-mate, so it was now easy to move a cot in or out! There was a door leading to the flat roof, and one to the hall, outside of which there was no privacy. We had a large living room and dining room, and the former contained the same leather chairs and tables we had before — our mess furniture that had travelled with us and was still in good condition. We also had the bar — very important to everyone. Our same mess sergeant, with the home sister and the stewards, set everything to right. The home sister served tea in the afternoons to anyone at home, and all officers making a visit, even if they did not know anyone but were hoping to make friends while on leave.

The entrance was on the corner of a side street, off the promenade along the Tiber. When we returned from work, we found two Canadian soldiers on guard at the iron gates near the sidewalk. Inside the gate were a few steps, and then a wide stone set of stairs leading to double doors that were never locked. The guards were on duty twenty-four hours a day, and guarded the side doors as well. In addition, all the windows had old rusty iron grills, not installed by the Army, but there for the little girls. We were very safe.

The food was the same, all dehydrated — ground beef, ground up potatoes, and cauliflower. Dinner was as usual, with Spam and bully beef (short for the French *boeuf bouilli* — "boiled meat"), either cold or cooked one way or another — sometimes in a "blanket" of some kind of pastry (in name only!). But there was always lots of good cheddar cheese and hard biscuits and bread. We did all right; we ate the rations of the Eighth Army, so we all had the same — except the Americans.

There were large, very old apartment houses behind our quarters, where someone was always singing operatic arias in Italian. Spaghetti was constantly being made outside on long wooden tables set up in a courtyard; it was rolled, cut into strips, and hung on lines.

Molly and I went shopping in our free time. In an American PX I bought myself some khaki silk panties, and a new necktie. The British officers' shop would not have had them.

Along the streets of Rome were small shops with huge iron shutter-type doors that were pulled down at night. Later, black market stalls were set up on the sidewalks along the river. Once, while taking a short cut to visit the expensive shops on the *Via Condotti*, near the famous Spanish Steps, I saw meat being sold; the carcasses were hanging, and I could see the feet — dog paws! The meat was served in restaurants as ham. I could not eat pink meat again, but could never tell my friends why, because they enjoyed it so much! It made me ill to see it served. It was usually offered on a small plate as hors d'oeuvres.

In Sicily, and now in Rome, I had severe bronchial coughs, and the Matron was quite sympathetic, advising me to go to the operating room every day and use the infrared lamp on my chest. This applied only when I was on night duty and the equipment was available. It really helped me, as there was certainly no cough syrup available, and my cough cleared up each time.

Some of our Roman Catholic nurses invited several small groups of nuns to the mess for dinner. They were very thin, almost emaciated. In return, the nurses asked the nuns to embroider the sheets they had brought with them from the hospital in Catania, as the nuns' handiwork was most beautiful. These lovely pure linen sheets were found in the hospitals both in Sicily and Italy, and many were used in the operating rooms. The air mattress given to me by an Air Force officer in Sicily had given out, so I took a couple of sheets of the heavy cotton double flanelette variety to use as a mattress on my cot. They made a very thick — and comfortable — mattress.

And when my bathing suit finally wore out in Rome, I took one of the linen sheets from the O.R. and made myself a two-piece bathing suit. I had to sew it by hand, but it turned out well.

CHAPTER FOURTEEN

Visiting the Sacred — and the Profane

One day I was ordered by the Matron to put my name on a "Command Party" list. Even though I had resolved never again to do this, the Matron could order us to go. This one was at the American Club in the Excelsior Hotel, and was sponsored by the Canadian Green Berets. These men were shock troops who had trained in the Florida swamps with the American Army. They were still attached to the Americans, so were allowed to use their hotels and clubs. A very tough crowd!

When we arrived we were taken upstairs where there was a vast array of bottles, promising a difficult kind of party to be caught up in. Before long I left the rooms when I had a chance, and went downstairs where I hoped to find someone I knew who would take me back to our mess. I had few hopes, because only Americans or those attached to the American armies were present. I crossed a small deserted dance floor into the lobby, where I ran into a friend I had met in England, but did not know was in Rome. He was with the British First Army, attached to the American Fifth Army, and had fought in the Battle of Anzio, which had drawn German troops from Cassino and helped make its defeat possible. His outfit was now camped in Cork Forest near the Lido, a very elite Italian beach area. The whole long beach had been heavily laid with land mines, but a large space had been cleared to make it safe to swim. Much to my relief, he drove me to my mess. The party would be one woman short, but hopefully it would not be noticed. I never heard that I was missed, but some nurses were peeved that I had not told them I was leaving, as they would have liked to have left with me. C'est la guerre!

Another nurse and I went sightseeing to St. Peter's, where a priest offered to guide us. At the end of the tour he hurried us down a side hall into a large room with a platform. The room was full of American officers. The priest kept telling us to hurry, if we wanted to see Pope Pius, but we did not believe him. He took us to the front of the room, and under the platform, where there were two Scottish officers from the Gordon Highlanders, more veterans of the Battle of Anzio. They were in their kilts, and had been brought in by the same priest.

We were all about to be received by the Pope, who was due to arrive at any minute! The Scots asked if we were Catholics. No, we were Presbyterians. So were they. We discussed whether or not we should kiss the Pope's ring if he offered his hand. We decided we would only bow. Then he was brought in, carried in a palanquin on the shoulders of four Swiss Guards. He stepped down on to the platform. He wore a long gown buttoned down the front, with a lovely shoulder cape made of a beautiful cream cashmere material. The first people he saw were the Scots in kilts and the two of us in our navy blue suits with Canada pins on our shoulders, below the platform and in front of him. The rest were all Americans. He appeared surprised, but welcomed us all to Rome. He spoke to the American officers — the other ranks were in another room — in Italian and English, as they were all supposed to have Italian ancestors!

The Pope walked down some steps, came straight towards us, and held out the hand with the beautiful ruby ring. The two Scots gave me a shove, and I almost fell in front of him. They wanted to see if I really intended to bow, and they would do the same. I bowed over his hand, and the other three did the same. He asked us where we were living and we told him. He knew only that the Americans had taken Rome — nothing of the Battle of Anzio where the Scottish Regiment had fought, or of the Canadians who had fought the Germans so hard on the road to Rome. The Americans were shouting, "Look this way, Pope", and "Over here, Pope." They all had cameras and were busy taking his picture.

The Pope's aide gave each of us a bronze medal, the size of a silver dollar. It had Romulus and Remus suckling the wolf on one side, and the Pope on the other. He had had it struck to commemorate the taking of Rome by the Americans. I think we may have been the only Canadians and Scots to receive it! Back at the mess, nobody would believe we had been received by the Pope, even though we showed them our medals. (Mine would one day be stolen from my home in Ottawa.)

On another occasion a priest took several of us to the vaults below St. Peter's. We walked down two floors of a small curved iron stairway to rooms filled with fabulous gold, silver and jewelled treasures, and costumes that popes had worn for centuries. They had been stored here to save them during the war. We saw wine goblets from the time of Charlemagne, encrusted with rubies, diamonds and emeralds, and we saw the most beautiful objets d'art, centuries old. Not many people were taken down to see them; I have never heard anyone else speak of the experience.

We often took visiting friends to St. Peter's, and also the Catacombs. There were nearly thirty in Rome, and they extended for hundreds of miles. We visited the Catacombs of St. Callixtus on the outskirts of the city. It prided itself on holding "the place of honour" amongst Roman Catacombs: "No other catacomb can claim such an outstanding number of illustrious martyrs and saints, amongst whom were some twenty Popes." However we were horrified to see, just inside the entrance, boxes full of the mutilated bodies of Fascists. Even worse was the sight of their boots lined up against the wall — with the feet still in them!

Later, we could not walk to work at the hospital because of the Italian uprisings. At stated times we went back and forth from our quarters to the hospital by transport, with armed guards. Local men were killing Fascists — or vice versa — and others who got in their way. Once, while I was serving as relief Night Supervisor, some allied soldiers who had been attacked by Fascists were brought into the hospital, but unfortunately many were too seriously injured to save.

An American nurse's body had been taken from the Tiber nearby, and I had to phone the American hospital — a sort of castle on one of the seven hills of Rome — and an American officer quickly appeared. I accompanied the body to their hospital in one of our ambulances, with the officer leading in his car. My ambulance driver was very worried about my going inside, and said if I was not out in ten minutes he would come in and look for me! I had to have my papers signed by the Officer Commanding, in return for the body.

That was the same day I witnessed the bartender in one of the hotel clubs make up a cocktail with cherry brandy, Italian cognac, and canned milk that some officers had contributed. They had asked him to make something "original." The canned milk was part of their rations, and they carried it with them because it was great to trade. They wanted a name for the cocktail, and decided to call it after the British General Harold Alexander; thus the "Alexander Cocktail" came into being. It was believed that since it contained canned milk, you could never become tipsy from drinking it!

One night our medical officers and nursing sisters were holding a dance, with a band, in the Nursing Sisters' Residence. I was late arriving, as I had just come off duty. The music was very good, and I was talking to someone when I heard, "May I have this dance?" Imagine my surprise to see "The Major" — the former private I had dated in Sicily! I thought Jessie must have asked him to the dance, but she hadn't; he had heard a rumour and, being in Rome, decided to come along. I thought someone would surely know him, but he just laughed. He was a wonderful dancer, with a great sense of humour, and he asked me to marry him while we were dancing! I asked him if he had taken lessons from Arthur Murray's Dance Company, and he said, "I taught them!" Later in the evening we were again dancing, and I suddenly noticed we were the only ones on the floor. The band stopped, there was applause, and he said, "I told you so!"

I will always remember another man, an American named Jimmy. He always seemed to have a twenty-four-hour leave — or a few days! In

Rome he would appear in a jeep, with a driver — always the same driver — and a "boot-locker", a metal box which fitted nicely on the floor. Jimmy was always certain that we were engaged, and would be married after the war. But he thought I was a bit short — although my hands were very nice! And my bones were very good — at least, the ones he could see. However, I was to wear my hair up on top of my head when I got out of the Army and we were married. It seemed I would have to change somewhat — although I would always be short!

A large number of German patients arrived after a battle north of Florence. They had been left behind by the German Army. Each man carried a postcard-sized slip of paper, one side of which was entitled "Safe Conduct" and had the same message in German and English:

> The GERMAN SOLDIER who carries this SAFE CONDUCT is using it as a sign of his genuine wish to give himself up. He is to be disarmed, to be well looked after, to receive food and medical attention as required, and is to be removed from the danger zone as soon as possible.

The other side was German only, and had two comments: "DIE ALLI-IERTEN SIND IN DEUTSCHLAND!" and "WOFUR VERTEIDIGST DU NOCH ITALIEN?"

As we had no room, the prisoners were put on stretchers in the courtyard, and looked after by their own people. They certainly didn't like us, and shouted at us as we crossed the courtyard to get inside. Symphony concerts were presented in the courtyard, for both staff and patients — including the Germans. There, in a former Fascist/Nazi academy, were now heard "O Canada" and "God Save the King."

Some of the German medical personnel worked for us on the wards, and one man assigned to me was very knowledgeable and a great help. He had been a university medical student, and owned the best array of surgical instruments I had ever seen. We treated him well; I gave him the same vitamins and mepacrine that we gave to patients.

He cried when he left; he wanted to give me a case of his instruments, but I refused.

The buildings and grounds of the Foro Mussolini, which was to have been the site of the 1940 Olympic Games, became a leave and recreation centre for American troops and the British attached to them. Officially it was designated "5th Army Rest Center." The food in the officers' dining room was always very good, with a dish of cherry jam and one of peanut butter on each table. While watching Americans eating both of these items with their pork chops, we were always astonished! You could not go in there unless you were with an American officer, or an Allied officer attached to the Americans.

Foro Mussolini was an amazing place. Swimming pools were located on top of each building. There was a long avenue lined with statues of the various sporting disciplines, and the stadium had tiered marble seats. The Canadians had a big sports meet there, that I was able to attend because I was on night duty. Then on 15 and 16 July I went to the "Allied Track and Field Championships", which involved both the Mediterranean and North African forces, and attracted an audience of 15,000 troops. The amount of organization that went into staging this must have been incredible. The program listed all competitors in every event. Musical accompaniment was provided by the Band of His Majesty's Grenadier Guards, the Band of the 245th Army Ground Forces (U.S.), and the Band of the 2nd Marrocan Division (France). As reported in **The Maple Leaf** on 17 July, "Canadian athletes Find Going Tough"; they had been "blacked out completely, failing to place among the first three in any one event." However, Lt.-Gen. E.L.M. Burns, the Canadian commander, had played a prominent part; he officially greeted the athletes and "personally congratulated each of the winners, presenting the first three in all events with handsome gold wrist watches." Two other events had already been held: The Allied Boxing Championships in Algiers, and the Theatre Championship for Basketball in Oran. Still to come was the Allied Swimming Championships in Rome the following month. I wondered how the military had found time to organize these events while fighting a war, but they were great morale boosters!

At the end of July the medical ward I was working on was quarantined for a week due to an outbreak of measles, and we could not admit or discharge any patients during that period. I had had measles as a child and was considered immune, so I stayed to work on the ward with the affected patients until we were considered free of it. I could come and go, but not the up-patients, who became bored. One day I found them leaning out the windows; they had tied their blue blankets together, hung them outside, and were selling them to a crowd in the street below! I had to call a sergeant to settle the matter.

My move to the opposite side of the courtyard to an amputation ward was a great change. The thirty beds were in a large classroom on the second floor, with an officers' ward across the hall. About ninety percent of the patients on my ward, and another downstairs, were amputees of one or both legs. The greater number had been caused by the explosion of land mines. We were equipped with one pair of crutches. We also had one tiny pressure stove, one kidney basin, one pair of forceps, and one bathroom. We used Dakin Solution, which is chloride of lime — a very old treatment — for wound compresses. We continued to inject penicillin directly into knee and shoulder joint wounds, but because it was so painful for the patients I mixed it with sterile local anaesthetic before injecting it.

We had to teach the amputee patients muscle exercises for an injured leg. They did them a prescribed number of times a day to keep the muscles supple, to be prepared for an artificial limb. The men were often depressed from the trauma of their injury. I always told them they would go back first to England, to a rehabilitation hospital, where they would get a new "tin" leg, and learn to walk with it before going back to Canada. I also told them about Douglas Bader, who had been stationed near us at Marston Green. After losing both legs, he was still allowed into the Air Force with two "tin" ones. When he became a prisoner of war the Germans took away a leg so he would stop trying to escape, and the RAF dropped him a replacement!

There were several German prisoners on the amputation ward, and they had been placed in beds in the centre of the room. The other patients liked to have them there so they could not escape. We treated the Germans as well as anybody with our short supply of penicillin. However, they were terrified of the penicillin being injected into their wounds, thinking they were being deliberately infected or poisoned, and would die. One officer of the German Elite Corps had a horrible shoulder wound, and was in a side room. He too thought he was being poisoned. He called us every name possible in German, and I finally had to ask the Medical Officer to evacuate him to a base hospital.

One day one of the patients complained of a swollen left wrist. He had a wound on the inside of the wrist that had not healed, so I boiled my little forceps and opened the wound. I saw something black. Not knowing what it could be, but knowing that the beginning of gangrene could be indicated, I probed and tugged, and emerged with half of a leather wristwatch strap! The patient had lost his watch when he received his leg wound after a mine exploded, and his wrist had been struck at the same time. Once the strap was removed, the wound healed nicely.

Earlier, the same patient had had his left leg amputated. He was taken to the Operating Room just before dinner. I was serving the meals, and had no way of keeping his dinner warm. The patients who were helping me urged me to eat it. It was fresh meat, and they insisted he would not want it when he came back. So I ate it. The patient returned, came out of the anaesthetic very quickly, and wanted his dinner! I had to confess that I had eaten it and there was nothing left. The poor man had to go hungry until supper time.

There was an outbreak of diptheria on this ward. When the first case was discovered, we all had to be inoculated. The staff had all been inoculated regularly, but I knew I could not take it, so I told the

Colonel, the hospital O.C., that I had been in close contact with diptheria when I was small. He knew what I meant, so I didn't have the inoculation. No one knew the story of my "inoculations" in Montreal, and I managed to get by without having any.

So again I was left on a ward that was quarantined because I was thought to be immune — this time from diptheria. There were to be no admissions, discharges or evacuations. The medical officers and nurses came and went, but the patients were confined. If a week passed and there were no further outbreaks, the quarantine would be lifted. The Medical Officer made daily rounds and examined throats while sitting on the patients' beds. We took weekly throat swabs from all the patients, as well as the medical officers and nurses. Then it was discovered that the M.O. was the carrier! A week later, the quarantine was lifted. During the enforced confinement the patients had little to do but play cards, but the Red Cross women produced needlepoint kits, and most of the patients worked on them. One of them gave his finished piece to me.

Sometimes, unexpectedly, ugly incidents could occur. The windows of the ward I was on were two floors up, and looked out over the street and the Tiber, where tragic events happened frequently. One day the patients called me to witness three bodies hanging by their heels out of the windows of the city jail next door. I could hardly believe it! They had been executed, and displayed there as a warning to Fascists. One body was that of a woman.

I was again on night duty on this ward, and a friend was on night duty downstairs. The patients had terrible nightmares, reliving their battles, as had been the case all through the time we were in the Mediterranean area. I heard about all their fears, and about the deaths of friends, all too real I thought. I shared an orderly with the downstairs ward, and one night he came running to me, saying the nurse there needed my help. I ran down and found an officer lying on the floor, with a bayonet in his hand ready to kill himself. He claimed he was Christ, and that he could kill himself and live again. We had a terrible struggle, but he finally gave up the weapon and we tied him up in a sheet.

He was evacuated the next day.

CHAPTER FIFTEEN

Fun at the Fair

When we came off night duty we were offered a week's leave. We could go to a leave hotel in Amalfi, just south of Naples, but my friend Molly and I decided we would rather go to the San Dominican Hotel in Taormina, Sicily, on the coast between Catania and Messina, and close to Mount Etna. I had been to Taormina for part of a day while in Sicily, but Molly had never been, having joined our outfit when we were in Cancello. However, she had heard about the beauty of the place. The San Dominican was off the main road and perched on the side of a cliff, at the bottom of which were lovely beaches. It had been first a monastery, then (like the Grand Hotel Etna where I had previously stayed), a German head-quarters, then British Headquarters, and finally a leave hotel. A very old part of it remained as it had been before the war. In addition to the hotel, there was an ancient Greek theatre in the area, which had been rebuilt by the Romans, and some other Roman ruins.

We could go as far as Naples with the others in the transport provided, and then try to hitch a ride to Catania from the airport, where we knew there were Air Force personnel. We went to the Air Force office in Rome, made inquiries, and were assured it was possible to get a plane from Naples. We decided to keep quiet about our arrangements so that the Matron, or others in authority, would not scuttle our plan.

When we arrived in Naples we told the driver and the other nurses that we were stopping there. We then went to the British Officers' Club, had tea, and asked how to get to the airport. We learned there was a transport that picked up air crew from various locations, and that it was at that moment parked outside the club! We were driven to the crew office at the airport, where we found a Mitchell bomber with two American pilots. They had been shopping in Malta for fruit and vegetables for their new mess, and were about to take off for Catania. They agreed to ferry us, and we clambered aboard. It was about 6 p.m. and the weather was good.

When we landed in Catania I was surprised to meet Air Force friends I had known, who were also just arriving. They took us to their mess, fed us, and found us a room in a guest house. I never did get into town to see if it had changed. However, there was certainly no change at the airport. It was all new to Molly.

The next day my friends gave us transport to Taormina. The road was good, and I could see our old hospital still standing on its hill. When we arrived at our destination, our friends promised to send transport for us when we were leaving, and even to fly us back to Caserta, familiar territory and close to Naples.

What a string of luck!

We found the San Dominican full, but were taken to a house used for overflow, although we had our meals at the hotel. The place was run by the British and was not expensive. There were lots of places for sightseeing, and there was transport to and from the glorious beaches, where we spent nearly all our days. We rented an umbrella, towels and flat chairs very cheaply, and there were several canteens where we could get refreshments. Every evening at dinner we met many old friends who were also on leave.

After a wonderful, relaxing vacation we were returned to Catania, flown to Caserta, and driven to Rome in an ambulance. We got back on time, no one questioned us, and we never told anyone where we had been. Certainly the Matron wasn't curious.

We worked hard and lived uncomfortably, but we had our moments!

Rome had become a dangerous place in which to live. People were often being beaten, and some killed and thrown in the river by riotous crowds. While we were walking in Rome, the Fascists would sometimes push us off the sidewalks. As a result of all this we were partially confined to barracks, and continued to be driven back and forth from work in jeeps or halfton trucks with armed guards.

I was crossing the front foyer of the hospital one day when two British soldiers were brought through the entrance by two of their friends. They were dying, as a couple of medical officers and myself went to help them. They were put on stretchers, but all we could do was give them injections to ease their pain. They were so mutilated that no one could do anything. It was a horrible sight to watch two healthy young men die, especially after they had survived the battles in Sicily and Italy, and perhaps before that in the North African desert. They had probably been on leave, enjoying life, when they were attacked by a mob. We assumed the attackers were Fascists, who seemed to hate both Allies and Germans alike.

Continuing to keep ourselves and our uniforms clean and presentable was difficult, and took much of our time. There was so little water with which to wash our clothes, and no iron to press them. There were as yet no detergents, so we used hand soap on our laundry. At a party, a British Army colonel, a Scot, said to me, "You must have grave problems washing your smalls." By this time I was familiar enough with his vocabulary not to be offended, because I knew he was talking about my underwear!

When patients came in without kits, there were no replacements available, so we had to scrounge. We had two Red Cross women in our unit, as well as others from the Salvation Army. It was better to go to the Salvation Army for socks, razors, etc., as they were glad to give to the soldiers and help them freely, whereas with the Red Cross we had to exchange worn out things for new ones.

In August 1944 the 1st Canadian Division, the U.S. Fifth Army, and the First British Army were near Florence. We heard that the buildings in the city had been spared, but nearly all the bridges were destroyed, with the exception of the *Ponte Vecchio*. Then we heard that the Canadians were in eastern Italy, and had taken Rimini. This city, part of which dated to 27 B.C., was reduced to rubble. 22 September was the last day of action for the Canadian Division, and they were relieved by New Zealanders. This was in the midst of very heavy fighting, and many casualties had been sustained. We heard rumours that we would be going to Rimini, but we found out that No. 1 CGH was to go instead, so we knew we would be staying in Rome. There were many rumours flying around, and we listened to them all!

Winter arrived, and with it the theatres were opening, which was wonderful — ballet, opera, plays — and they were always sold out. I enjoyed going to the ballet best; in Montreal we had been treated to the Ballet Rousse at His Majesty's Theatre at least once a year. The theatres in Rome had retractable roofs, to air them out after a performance! **Ali Baba and the Forty Thieves** was put on as a pantomime in a local theatre by the men of the Royal Artillery Regiment. It was very professionally produced and performed.

On Christmas Eve the staff sang carols in the central square below the wards, helped by a group of English soldiers who were visiting. Several Canadian soldiers came to my ward to visit others from their regiment; they all had at least two bottles with them when they arrived, so it was quite a noisy affair! We officers cooked and served dinner on Christmas Day to the patients and other ranks. For the occasion twenty turkeys were transported from No. 1 Echelon to the hospital, but on the way six were stolen by children, some of whom had mastered the art of stealing from moving trucks. Besides the limited supply of roast turkey, Christmas dinner consisted of fruit salad, mashed potatoes and giblet gravy, creamed corn and peas. For "afters" there was Christmas pudding with brandy sauce and mincemeat pie, all washed down with plenty of beer. The beer, which came in twenty litre bottles, was made in Rome by the English for the benefit of all Allied forces. Every ward had its own decorations and Christmas tree, and even bunches of mistletoe were hung around the hospital. Our Christmas festivities were so successful that they were reported in Canadian newspapers, along with the news, "Maj. Glen Miller, famous American band leader, is missing in action."

On Boxing Day, the staff had our dinner. As officers, we were charged extra mess fees for our meal — 700 lira — which we thought was too much. But it was an exceptionally good one — no dehydrated food!

The year 1945 opened with more rumours — we heard that all Canadian forces would be moving into central Europe. In the meantime, soldiers were being admitted to the hospital with alcohol poisoning from Italian-made alcohol. Home brew could be very dangerous, and many died from it. Heaven knew what they made it from, but it was very available; you were offered it in many an officers' mess, mixed with lime juice to give it a better flavour. I never liked it and rarely drank it, but it was always easy to drink lime juice if they offered nothing else.

The weather was very cold, and although we had no heat, we did have electricity. We bought small electric one-ring burners, which we hooked to the light sockets in the ceiling, so we could cook in our rooms with food purchased on the black market — eggs, bacon, and tomatoes. We also bought an electric iron for our clothes.

Archbishop Villeneuve arrived at the hospital to visit the patients of the Royal 22nd Regiment, 1st Division — the "Van Doos." Being from Montreal and able to speak some French, I was asked by the Matron and Colonel to be on duty. I told them I had met the Archbishop before, and that he spoke and understood English, but preferred French. When he arrived, he brought me a message from my friends in Three Rivers, Quebec! During his visit, we all spoke English.

On 17 February we heard more rumours about moving, this time to England or France, by boat. There were now few Canadians in Rome, as they had moved ahead of us. We packed part of the ward and our personal gear. We were told to wear khaki pants, boots, and canvas gaiters. Whenever the order was to wear our gaiters, we knew we were going by ship. On 5 March we moved from the hospital to the Chateau Laurier, where we were two to a room in a very cold, unheated hotel. However, we never grumbled seriously, as this was sometimes our way of life.

Rome was particularly lovely in the spring of 1945. The flowers on sale at the Spanish Steps were gorgeous, and were displayed all up and down the sides of the wide staircases. Flower girls were selling baskets of lovely Parma violets, with their gorgeous perfume, outside the hotels. A friend who took me out to lunch bought me a whole basket of them afterwards.

We were allowed to go wherever we liked, but not alone. One morning Molly and I went to the American Hotel Excelsior, which was now more or less open to all officers. There we had a Turkish bath, surrounded by Italian prostitutes! On the way back to the Chateau Laurier, we were unaware that we were about to have one of the worst experiences of our lives. We suddenly became caught up in a mob of Italians in a piazza, and were shoved to the centre, where an Italian man was being held on the ground. The mob was shouting and screaming, "Fascist! Fascist!" While we stood there, one man with a knife tore off the victim's top clothes, and stabbed him. The assailant then cut out his heart, while he was alive and screaming, and while others continued to hold him down. Finally, the heart was held aloft on the end of the knife. We were stunned and horrified! It was terrible standing there in the front row, hemmed in by these men, not knowing what might happen to us. Then we were shoved violently out of the crowd, and we ran away as fast as we could.

The crowd had known who we were from our uniforms, and from the CANADA badges on our shoulders. I believe they had wanted us to witness the incident; we were still the enemy to the Italians, and they just wished to show us what they could and would do. When we reached the hotel, everyone knew by the looks on our faces that something horrible had happened, and we were given a drink to settle us down so we could tell our story. After that, we were not allowed out without a male escort.

We paid mess fees of 45 lira a day while at the Chateau Laurier, but...we had an egg for breakfast! Our mess sergeant came to me one day to ask a favour. He started by saying, "I know you don't have much money to take out of Italy with you..." He knew my financial status, because I had gone shopping and spent all my lira! He ran the mess, and was supposed to know everything, like a sergeant-major. He heard us talking in the mess, so he was aware of who our friends were, how much our mess bills were, how much we drank — and how many lira we had. His problem was that he had been playing poker while we were waiting to leave, and had been winning, with the result that he had too much money. There was a limit to the amount of Italian currency we could take out of the country. So I agreed to allow some of it to travel with me.

Our hospital was to leave Rome for Belgium, but before we left, Jimmy — my "fiancé" — came to the city on one of his frequent twenty-four-hour passes. After dinner he told me he had a surprise for me to remember him by — that is, until we met again. We drove south through the city until we arrived at a small fair. It had a merry-go-round and a ferris wheel. We stopped. There was a little old man beside the merry-go-round, and I was introduced to him. Jimmy, it seemed, had met him before. In fact, Jimmy had persuaded the man to run the fair for one whole evening just for the two of us. My surprise! And with the lights and the music. The horses on the merry-go-round were beautiful, moving up and down to the music. The old man spent the evening running both the merry-go-round and the ferris wheel, just for us! He would stop the ferris wheel when we were at the top, so we could look at the stars. Such fun! Such a lovely memory!

Sadly, before I left Rome I wrote to Jimmy to try to tell him we were not meant to marry. I really could never change myself as he wanted. I received letters begging me to reconsider. I never learned if his regiment stayed in Italy after I left, or returned to the United States. In fact, I never saw Jimmy again.

Part Eight — Up to Belgium

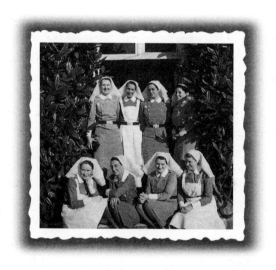

CHAPTER SIXTEEN

And It's Farewell to "The Major"

Entries from my diary:

12 March — Left early by ambulance in our khaki battle dress, jacket, pants, gaiters, and boots. It was very uncomfortable driving the long distance to Naples. Arrived at 3:30 p.m. and went to a British Sisters' Transient Camp, a big, bare old building. We were housed on the second floor where there were beds and nails on the walls to hang our clothes. Camp is on the summit of the city with a spectacular view of the harbour. Orders to leave next day.

14/15 March — Boarded the *Indapura of Liverpool* in the harbour. Over 2,000 troops on board. Had to share a cabin with thirteen others. As we were going down to lunch one of the officers coming up told us there was steak on the menu: "Horse meat, but damn good, and all you want to eat." We moved out at 4 p.m. Amazingly I met an officer from where I had grown up in New Brunswick. What an odd way to meet and recognize each other! We were on deck that day and all the next. Saw schools of porpoises. We passed between Corsica and Sardinia.

16 March — Docked in Marseilles at 10 a.m. Had lunch on board (ham on large white buns) and disembarked about 2 p.m. On shore went to an American hospital where there were coal fires in every room. Such luxury! We are to fly out tomorrow. Very warm.

17 March — Flew from Marigana Airport in a Dakota which had been used for paratroopers. There was no heat and the flight took four hours, passing over the Alps where we became colder still. My feet were frozen and very painful. We landed at Sabina Airport in Brussels, and then to Ghent, where we set up in a horse stable with marble stalls and floor — a Horse Palace! We each had a stall in which to set

our cots. We were told we could have ten days leave in England. We had to volunteer to go and four of us will be leaving in the morning on a 7 a.m. flight for Croydon Airport. No one is allowed to go to Paris. Changed billets, and are now at No. 2 Canadian General Hospital, thirty to a room. Using our canvas cots again.

18 March — Up at 6 a.m. and caught the plane after the driver had driven us around for hours looking for it. It was a one and a half hour flight to Biggin Hill Airport, where we boarded a bus for London. Reported in to a women's transient residence that belongs to the Swan & Edgar's department store on Regent Street, but as we could only stay there for forty-eight hours, we went instead to the Nursing Sisters' Club (Mr. Weston's), now under Red Cross management. Exhausted. Told they had no rooms for us. We went to the Knights of Columbus Club and accommodation has been found for us at the Savoy Hotel, but it won't be available until tomorrow. So we will spend the night back at the residence. Went to see a play. London full of Canadians on leave; it seems the entire 1st Division is here.

In fact, everyone — troops and nursing sisters — from Italy had been sent on leave to London. We knew many of these people from Sicily and Italy, of course, and exchanged news and opinions of where we were going next. Was it to Canada?

We all needed money, so I went to the Bank of Montreal where I had my account. I intended to draw out some for myself and enough to lend to a nurse who for some reason had no money. The bank was full of officers, and I was thankful that no one recognized me, because as we approached the teller, who knew me well, she cried, "Sister Carter! It's good to see you! Your account is wonderful!" Everyone in the bank laughed and laughed. I was glad they were strangers! I have never forgotten her or that day! She had good reason to say this, because when I had been in England before I was always going to her to advance me money from my next month's pay to cover my hotel bills. Now, when I wanted to draw out what she considered a large sum, she said, "Just when you have a tidy amount in your account, you are drawing it out!" Everyone laughed again. They all thought she was glad to see me safe, after, as she said, "about two years" away in the war. I always thought of her as "Pearl White" of the silent movies, who I had seen when I was very small, with her ropes of beads hanging and jingling with each movement. She had always been trying to get me to save my money, in order to have a good balance in my bankbook. Now, because as a junior officer I had only been allowed to write chits for a limited amount each month outside of England, I had plenty of cash left over in the bank.

While in London we went to various clubs and shows every night: **Chin Chin Chow** was still playing, and a Canadian performance of **Meet the Navy** at the Strand Theatre was very good. I had bought a lovely green suede vest which I wore to **Meet the Navy**, and afterwards we went backstage to meet some of the dancers and the nursing sister from the Navy who was travelling with the show to look after them. (When I moved to Ottawa after the war, I met a high school teacher who had been in the Navy and was a "hoofer" in that production.) We went to a theatre on Lower Regent Street to see Gertrude Lawrence. At the interval someone said that the star had just received news her son had been killed. Yet she courageously went on with the show.

I went down by train to see some English friends in the village of Wonersh, near Guildford, and I stayed overnight. While stationed at Dorking, I had walked part of the "Pilgrim's Way" with them, starting at Guildford. This was a prehistoric trackway which had been used by the Romans, and later by medieval pilgrims travelling from Winchester to Canterbury to visit the tomb of St. Thomas à Becket. After that I visited Basingstoke, to see everyone I knew at the Canadian Neurological Hospital.

We gave up our rooms at the Savoy because we were to fly back to Europe that afternoon. But at the Auxiliary Transport Service Club we learned that we were to return the next day. So we had to find beds for the night. We went to the Strand Palace Hotel, which had been "out of bounds" to Canadians in the early years of the war. But not now. The next day we reported again to our air transport, and were told, "Maybe tomorrow." Instead of flying, I bought some books and managed to get two pairs of stockings at the Canadian Women's Auxiliary Corps Headquarters — two shillings and sixpence a pair. No flying the next day, but we were told that we would definitely leave on the next, a Friday. We duly caught transport to Biggin Hill after calling Air Headquarters to confirm our flight. We flew with several other officers and arrived in Brussels, where we took a train to Ghent. We were back at No. 2 CGH, and once more were thirty to a room.

Sunday, 1 April. We went to an Easter church service in the city. Upon our return, a padre was waiting to take me to see my brother Bill, who had been in the Second Front. We were glad to see each other, although he looked awfully tired and older — and extremely thin. But didn't we all! He had volunteered with a friend in his artillery unit to run railway engines in Belgium, France and Holland, carrying supplies and the wounded. They had taken courses in England, and gone over early in the attack on the Second Front. It was a hazardous job, as sometimes railway bridges were bombed, and even the trains. Bridges were out, and new bridges were put in — but in the dark of night. The going was bad, with no light except when they had to open the firedoor, which was very dangerous as it could be seen from a great distance. Bill was due to go back to Canada soon.

Several of us got permission and passes to go to Brussels. No women were allowed in the Army Officers' Club there, so we went to the Allied Officers' Club instead. The people of Brussels were very friendly towards Canadians, and we became real tourists. The city was lovely, and the parts we saw were untouched by the war. There was a fine central square — such beautiful old buildings! Every structure in the square was magnificent, and extremely old. The eleventh-century Hotel de Ville was City Hall, and the most attractive and largest of the buildings. There was an order of nuns who lived in Brussels, in a large house and two rows of tiny cottages on either side of a driveway. These nuns were famous for their lace, and sat outside the cottages on their little pillows with their shuttles in their laps, making lace and selling it. (I would return five years later to find the city the same, except that the pastries were even richer and there was more handmade lace.)

I was taken to Mons, where there was an impressive monument to the First World War. The trenches were everywhere, and very well preserved. We went to First World War cemeteries — rows and rows of grave stones all the same, and the same distance apart, with flags from each country.

I was in for a big surprise while stationed in Ghent. I was on a sidewalk watching a Canadian Army unit marching down the street, when suddenly I noticed one of the privates waving his arm to attract my attention.

It was "The Major"!

I would not see him again.

Part Nine — Further up to England

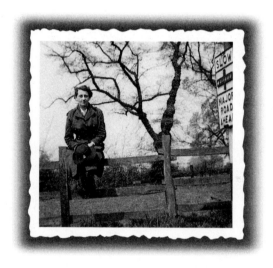

CHAPTER SEVENTEEN

Good Morning, Mother!

O
n 7 April I was told I would be returning to Canada, which I had expected as the rumour had been around for awhile. But to be suddenly told I was leaving was a great shock. However, I was not told precisely when I would be on my way, so it was like living in a vacuum. You were leaving good friends you had been with for a long while, and with whom you had been through good times and hard times; it was like losing your family. Being sent out into civilian life, into a crowd of strangers, or even people you knew but hadn't seen in a long while, was frightening, as was the expectation of freedom. We hadn't made our own decisions since going into the Army!

In the meantime we went sightseeing, on trains which had wooden slatted seats. We visited Bruges, a lovely old city, where another Canadian General Hospital was located. While in Bruges we had steak with an egg on top, a Belgian specialty. The name "Bruges" suggested "the place of bridges", and it was almost untouched by the war. Canals wound among the houses, and trees in their gardens hung over into the canals. A priest showed us around the huge Basilica of Notre Dame. Everything had been hidden from the enemy, but was now being put back in place. We saw Michelangelo's "Virgin and Child", a white statue which was the only work by the artist to leave Italy during his lifetime. We also viewed an amazing relic — a small white bone in a jewelled container with a glass top. A religious procession was held each year, during which the relic was said to bleed. I could see a dark spot by the relic, which was said to be blood. As to the Belgians themselves, it was rumoured amongst the military that they were on either side — whichever was winning — and that they had both German and Allied flags ready to put out.

Before we left for England a Canadian officer I met in the Medical Officers' Mess asked me if I had been to Dunkirk, and if not, I should see it. He wanted to take me, so we went in a jeep and visited what remained of the famous docks. I'm not sure I was glad I saw it, as I had seen so much like it in Sicily and Italy, although the officer thought there was no such devastation in those places.

We were all ordered to return to the hospital in Ghent on 13 April. The next day we did not leave for England as expected, but instead went by lorry to visit the Peace Memorial in Vimy. Like everywhere we visited, it was not a long distance from our hospital, which was a mile from the coast and sixteen miles from Ostend.

Things were getting worse. There were sixty nursing sisters living in a ward, with the result that it was impossible to sleep. We had few patients, so there was little work to do, and we seldom needed to go on duty. We wanted to go on leave to Paris, but were refused. Our mess was small, and was located in an old hotel close to an English-style cottage, which was the Medical Officers' Mess. There was no shortage of champagne and cherry brandy in their cellar! Finally, I was able to get some sleep when I moved to a bed in the hotel; the sister who normally used it was on night duty. We were told that General Rommel had stayed in the cottage while his troops were training on the hard sands nearby, before going to Africa.

There were about thirty of us from No. 5 CGH, from various medical fields, who were to return to Canada. We would go first to England, and I left with thirteen other nursing sisters on 24 April. After great leave-takings at the Medical Officers' Mess, we arrived at Ostend, where replacement nurses had recently arrived from England. Some would stay in Belgium, others would travel to France and Holland. Our Colonel and Matron accompanied us as far as the boat to see us off. The rumour was true: "First over, first back." We had been the first nursing sisters overseas, and we would be the first tranported back to Canada. And Mr. Mackenzie King had said that all nursing sisters would go back First Class!

We sailed at 2 p.m. for the trip across the Channel, on a boat which had participated in the Dunkirk evacuation, and still bore the scars. Lunch was at 5 p.m. — Spam and bread! The weather was cool, and the crossing smooth. We were issued blankets, and assigned to wooden bunks in a large cabin. In the morning we sailed up the Thames, past many sunken ships with only their masts visible above water.

At 11 p.m. we arrived at Tilbury Docks, where a lorry picked us up to take us to Bramshott, via Aldershot. After a miserable trip we arrived exhausted at 4 p.m. There were now eighty-five of us for "repatriation to Canada." We were ushered into a large barrack room in one of the old No. 15 CGH buildings, and given bunks. They were three-tiered and iron, and I was in a top one, more comfortable than a lower. I saw many friends who had arrived before me. The Matron gave us a set speech — we were allowed to go where we wished, but we had to sign papers, pack, and leave everything ready to be moved for us.

I made several day trips to different towns, including Brighton. A party of us went for a day by train. British trains were wonderful, and not expensive. In Brighton we could skate on rented skates and shop in the many antique stores. We walked along the boardwalk by the sea, and would sometimes see a convoy going by on the way to or from Canada, the U.S. or Ireland. I went back to see my friends at Guildford and East Grinstead. A few of us went to London for the day, wearing our navy blue suits and hats. Our uniforms were a bit bedraggled and needed pressing.

Back in Bramshott, we learned that VE Day was to be the next day — the war was over! We decided to go to London again, to celebrate, and we booked into the Canadian Sisters' London Club. We found the streets fairly quiet, until we caught up to the crowds going down The Mall towards Buckingham Palace. There, on the balcony, we saw the King, the Queen, and the rest of the Royal Family. Eventually, Mr. Churchill appeared, giving the Victory sign. I was beside the Victoria and Albert Memorial when suddenly I got separated from my friends. An English soldier lifted me up and put me on a ledge where there was a stone lion, and from there I was able to look out over the crowd and spot them. Eventually my friends saw me, and the soldier lifted me down and took me to them. I was nearly suffocated, and felt awfully lost in such a crowd, even though I knew how to get back to the Club. At night, it seemed all of London was floodlit.

We got back to the base on time, tired and footsore, as we were not used to walking so much on hard pavements. We were told we were in "Draft No. 155", and were confined to barracks as of 1800 hours. We could not leave the buildings. We washed and ironed our clothes, and arranged for the paymaster to transfer our bank accounts to Canada — the last thing to do.

On Thursday, 10 May, we left Bramshott at 9:30 a.m. Colonel Agnes Neill, Matron-in-Chief, gave us a pep talk, saying that we would be travelling back to Canada in comfort, First Class all the way! (We wondered later whether she knew how we were really going to travel!) However, as English war brides and their babies were also to be passengers, we would each have to work one shift in the baby clinic on board ship.

We boarded the train at Bramshott, slept in our seats, and arrived at Liverpool at 11 a.m. We had a long wait on the dock, and sat playing cribbage — waiting, always waiting! We embarked at noon, and as we had no backpacks it was an easy embarkation. The nursing sisters were located in two cabins on the bottom deck, C Deck. There were thirty in one cabin, and I was with fifty-four others who were allocated to a big cabin in the hold. The whole deck vibrated, and we could feel and hear the engines. So much for Miss Neill's speech about First Class treatment!

Again we were met by a host of three-tiered steel bunks and again I had a top bunk, complete with ladder, this time against a wall, which hopefully would prove comparatively cool and quiet. There were two bathrooms ("heads"), and always the floors were swimming in water. There were nine hundred brides and babies on the ship, all in First and Second Class — incidentally filling our reserved First Class accommodations! There were very few male officers and men, and they were located in another part of the lower deck. There were stewards and stewardesses, but they were not for us — we were on our own! Hourly information messages over the intercom for the mothers and babies added to the chaos and confusion. Two concessions had been granted us: we could use the sun deck on A Deck, where the mothers and babies were not allowed to go, and we had the senior officers' meal times by ourselves, except for several male officers, one of whom had his war bride with him. And oh yes, we were also allowed to spend our money in the ship's shop!

I took my shift in the medical room with the same pediatrician I had met as we evacuated our Casualty Clearing Station at Dorking. As I went in to work, I greeted him with, "Good morning, Mother, and how is Baby today?" It was good to work again with someone from the Royal Victoria Hospital.

We picked up our convoy in the Irish Sea, and had a sunny and calm voyage all the way home.

Part Ten — And Back to Canada

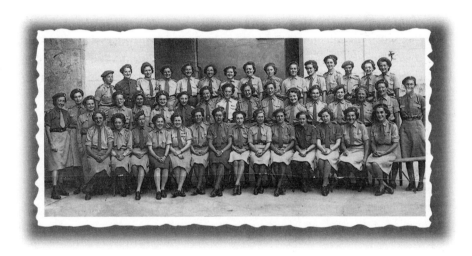

CHAPTER EIGHTEEN

It's String-pulling Time!

O ur ship arrived in Halifax Harbour on 23 May 1945. The Canadian Army Commanding Officer came on board with his staff, and over the intercom called a parade for all returning officers and ranks. It was held in the big First Class Salon. No war brides were allowed in!

Another sister and I decided to ask the C.O. for leave, to go directly to our family homes in the Maritimes instead of reporting to Headquarters in Montreal. We were very surprised to find him so agreeable. He gave us First Class tickets home, which would also take us from there to Montreal, after two weeks leave! I was taken by a Red Cross worker to the Halifax railway station and put on a train to Saint John, New Brunswick. I had a Pullman reservation and slept on the train. Arriving the next morning in Saint John, I was met by another Red Cross worker, who had come specially to pick me up. She was the sister-in-law of my younger sister, and she took me to her home. They were expecting me, because my name was on her list of war repatriots. I phoned my home in Woodstock, so they would meet my train the next day. Then I was served fresh shad for dinner; someone had gone to the market to get it especially for me. I stayed overnight.

The next morning, 24 May, I caught the train to McAdam Junction, to catch another train north to Woodstock. McAdam Junction is depicted on a Canadian one-dollar stamp; at one time it was very important, with trains travelling to and from St. Stephen, Fredericton, Saint John, Boston, New York, Montreal, and up the Saint John River Valley to Woodstock and on to Edmundston in northern New Brunswick. Private cars would be attached to the regular passenger trains, including many owned by people going to St.-Andrews-by-the-Sea.

My train was the last one out that day, as it always was. I arrived home at 9 p.m., and was met by all the family.

My older sister Eva and her son had arrived from Halifax; her two young daughters were already in Woodstock visiting my mother. Eva's husband, Commander Kingsmill, was now stationed in Halifax on harbour duty — no more convoying for him. I had no civilian clothes, except a cotton summer dress my mother had bought for me. So a week later Eva and I decided I needed some clothes, and we went to Montreal to shop for a few days. I used the travel warrant given to me by the C.O. on the ship. I bought a lovely wool red suit at the Jaeger shop, and a dark red linen two-piece dress with large red wooden buttons. It was wonderful to be able to wear other colours than the navy blue of the uniform I had on, and had been wearing for five years.

I had to go to Army HQ at the Sun Life Building, to get another travel warrant to New Brunswick and back to Montreal. I still had part of my two weeks left, and the officer in charge gave me another week's leave, which was very nice! He was surprised at my long service overseas. My sister and I returned to Woodstock, and a week or so later I reported for duty, again at HQ in Montreal. There the same officer who had inducted me into the Army met me! I asked if I could be discharged, and he replied that no nursing sisters were allowed to be discharged — they would all be needed for the sick and wounded returning soldiers. "Besides," he said, "you are too thin!" He told me I was to report for duty at the Queen Mary Veterans' Hospital on Queen Mary Road, where I would find the food very good, especially the Sunday desserts! He provided transport for me to the hospital, where I reported to the Matron — she had been Assistant Matron at No. 1 CGH when I first arrived in England. There I learned that my application for retirement from the Army had been "frozen." I had been denied.

I was assigned to a room in a building next door. I went on duty the next day, but I knew I wouldn't be staying. I would get my discharge myself, some way and soon! There were no medical officers or nurses

I knew, and few from overseas. And none of the patients were familiar. They were up-patients, and there was very little to do. It was boring. I felt out of place, with my cotton uniforms old and faded after nearly five years of wear overseas.

I planned to get a weekend off and visit Ottawa. I had been invited by my sister's mother-in-law, Lady Kingsmill, and I knew she could — and would — help me. She was the widow of Admiral Sir Charles Kingsmill, First Admiral of the Canadian Navy in World War One. I was allowed Saturday afternoon and Sunday off, and told to report back at 7 a.m. Monday morning. I found my sister Eva and her three children there before me. My sister told me she had once seen me in a newsreel at a movie theatre; I was struggling up the gangplank of a ship, laden down with my full kit, leaving England. She had never mentioned it before.

Eventually I told my sister and Lady Kingsmill my problem of leaving the Army. They solved it immediately. It seemed a General Mckenzie had been to lunch the day before, and would be just the one to go to. He had told them he had met me in London. I knew it wasn't me, but it could have been Sister Grace Carter, also of No. 1 CGH. As for me, I knew only one top brass — Brigadeer Turner, a friend of my father. His younger brother had been Commander of St. Helen's Island, Montreal, which was for prisoners-of-war — even Canadians, including Montreal's Mayor Houde.

It was decided that on my next trip to Ottawa Lady Kingsmill would get me an appointment with General Mckenzie. I returned two weeks later and it had been arranged. I went to his office, and found him very cordial. He phoned Quebec Army HQ at Longueil, where I would need an appointment to go for my discharge. The General said to the Officer Commanding, a colonel, "I have a nursing sister here in my office just back from five years overseas. She is at the Queen Mary Hospital in Montreal. Give her her discharge at once." It was a wonderful feeling to know I would be out of the Army soon, but I never dreamt it would happen the next day!

I went back to the hospital for duty Monday morning. The phone rang — the call was for me to report at once to the Matron and Colonel in the latter's office. I knew what it was about and hurried down, hoping they wouldn't be able to stop my discharge. I saluted and stood at attention. They were both very angry that I had gone over their heads to General Mckenzie, and had not even let them know what I intended to do. But thank goodness, a colonel could not question a general's orders!

They gave me transport to report to Longueil at once, and to report back to them. At Longueil the staff were very glad to help me, telling me I had the longest service overseas of any veteran who had yet applied for discharge. I was to receive extra pay for service in Canada, and more for overseas. Altogether, the Army now owed me two thousand and sixty-two dollars and fifty cents. So again the extra pay was considerable to me, and the most they had paid any veteran at Longueil so far. I was given a cursory physical examination by a doctor, I was weighed, and then I was given warm congratulations and a booklet entitled **Back to Civil Life.** My transport waited for me.

Later I would receive a "Certificate of Service Issued to Officers and Nursing Sisters", indicating I had been "appointed to Commissioned Rank in the Canadian Army (Active)" on 28 October 1940, and "was Struck Off the Strength" on 10 August 1945. It listed four of my medals: "1939-45 Star; Italy Star; Defence Medal; Canadian Volunteer Service Medal and Clasp." There was no mention of the medal awarded for serving in North Africa.

I reported back to the Matron. I was told in no uncertain terms to pack, take my trunk, and leave at once! Such an unpleasant — and mean — dismissal. "No one overseas ever did anything like that," I told her. "I will pack, but I will leave my trunk to be picked up later. When I know where I'm going, I will then send for it." I saluted and left.

When I finished packing, I wondered where I would go. Everyone I knew outside the Army was working. Then I thought of Dr. and Mme. Brault at their cottage on Ile Perrault, and decided to visit them. I had known them for many years, and the doctor always said he had two daughters — their real daughter Jeanne, and myself. Very close friends, Jeanne and I had been in training at the RVH in the same class. Jeanne had volunteered for war service as I had, but was rejected; she had been born in France, and was still a French citizen, as her parents had never taken out Canadian citizenship for her, believing it occurred automatically.

I took a train to Ste. Anne de Bellevue, west of Montreal. When I got off with my small suitcase, there were several cars lined up at the station platform. I saw one man standing by his car and I thought, "Good, there is a taxi." I went to him and asked if he would take me to Dr. Brault's cottage on Ile Perrault. He certainly looked me over; I thought he had probably never seen anything like my nursing sister's navy suit and hat before. I had not bothered to change, as I wanted to catch the train. Slowly he answered that he would take me "as far as the Four Seasons Hotel." I remembered the hotel, and thought I might find another taxi there, as it was more than a mile walk to the cottage.

I got in his car, and he took me to the hotel. I asked how much the fare was but he would not accept any money, and just said, "No charge." There was no other taxi available, so I walked off down the road, turned left on to a side road past a few cottages, and reached the Braults' at the end.

Mme. Brault was at home, and overcome to see me at the door. Jeanne, who was now working in the main operating room at the RVH, had told her I was back in Canada, but knew nothing about my going to see them. Dr. Brault was at Queen Mary Veterans' Hospital in St. Anne's, and would be home for lunch soon. I was to call Jeanne to let her know where I was, and that I needed a place to live. The doctor came in laughing his head off, but very glad to see me. He knew I was there; the "taxi driver" — who was actually the owner of the hotel — had phoned and told him he had a visitor, in what looked like a uniform! He also said I had taken him for a taxi driver, he had taken me to the hotel, and then let me walk the rest of the way. But he hadn't taken any money. Dr. Brault told him he should have taken me to the cottage, as I was just back from the war after nearly five years away with the 1st Division.

A few days later, Jeanne called and told me there was a room vacant in the apartment where she rented a room with kitchen privileges, and that she had reserved it for me. We would be four Royal Victoria nurses together! However, they were working, and I would now try to find something to do. My new home was a large red brick building on McArthur Street in Montreal, a few blocks from the RVH and near McGill University. I unpacked my trunk at once and, since I would be wearing civilian clothes, put away my uniforms.

I planned to visit the Superintendent of Nurses at the RVH, and also the one at the Neurological Building, Dr. Penfield's domain, to apply for a job. But before I had a chance to do this, I was walking down University Street to shop when I heard my name spoken behind me. I stopped, turned around, and heard again, "Miss Carter!" I recognized the woman almost at once, and was surprised she knew it was me. It was Miss Marion Lindenbergh. When I had first entered training at the RVH as a "probie" (the name given to a nurse-in-training before you were approved and received your "cap"), for six months we lived on Peel Street in the mansion given by J.K.L. Ross to the hospital. Miss Lindenbergh lived on the third floor — she was one of the two chaperones — and I came to know her well. She was a graduate of the Montreal General Hospital, and was now head of the School of Nursing at McGill University.

We had a chat on the sidewalk, and then she asked me to go with her to a large house nearby, which contained the McGill School of Nursing. Miss Lindenbergh introduced me to Miss Matheson, her assistant, as a new student in the Public Health Course! However, I explained that I did not have the money for fees. Miss Lindenbergh told me that the Government would pay them, and give me a living allowance as well because I was a war veteran. I had failed to read the **Back to Civil Life** booklet given to me upon my discharge at Longueil, which contained such information. I quickly made up my mind and agreed; I had made important spur-of-the-moment decisions before! My future had been changed by another chance meeting, which had resulted in my transfer to Algiers. And now, meeting Miss Lindenbergh on University Avenue had led to my enrollment in the Public Health Course.

I made many friends, enjoyed the work, and graduated in Public Health Nursing from McGill University. I then entered a three-month internship with the Victorian Order of Nurses, discovering that it had been founded in 1894 by Lady Isabel Aberdeen, wife of the Earl of Aberdeen, a former Governor General of Canada. I worked for the VON in Montreal, with families and unwed mothers, counselling them on their health and personal problems. Later I heard of a position as a public health nurse with the Collegiate Board of Ottawa. I went there for an interview, and was accepted. I was sorry to leave Montreal, but found I enjoyed living in Ottawa.

I soon became Supervisor of twenty-four high schools, each with its own public health nurse. On one memorable occasion, my experiences with malarial patients in North Africa would stand me in good stead. Our medical officer was very upset about a patient he had in hospital — a small boy. The child was running a very high temperature and experiencing severe chills. I talked with him about the boy's condition, and asked the doctor if he had been out of Canada, or was from a foreign country. Yes, he was. So I quickly diagnosed and told the doctor, "It is malaria; you should phone and get the intern to take a blood smear during the chill — and look for the microparasite." He phoned, gave the order, and went back himself to the hospital. He returned in a short time to tell me it was malaria, and to congratulate and thank me for my diagnosis, which had saved the child's life. So I hadn't forgotten my war experience with malaria patients, although in

El Arrouch we diagnosed them with one microscope and four glass slides! Nor did we have a medical officer to tell us to start the medication; it was a standing order.

In 1966 I was asked by Miss Isabelle Black, Head of Public Health Nursing for Ontario, to attend the University of Toronto to complete my degree in nursing, and then teach in their School of Nursing at the university. I really did not want to teach, or to live in Toronto, but asked if I could take the one-year post-graduate course in Administration in Public Health. I got a leave of absence from the school board to move to Toronto, and Miss Black kindly made arrangements for the Public Health Department to pay my fees and provide a living allowance. Upon completion of the course, I returned to my former position in Ottawa.

When Canada and Russia were building the Aswan Dam on the Nile River in Egypt, I was asked by the chief engineer of a Canadian engineering firm to accept the job of Matron of a hospital being built at Aswan for Canadian workers on the project. However, I did not want to go into a foreign land alone, even though there were Canadians there. Besides, I have always believed that Canada is by far the most pleasant country in the world to live in.

I refused the position, and have lived in Ottawa ever since.

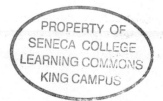